ANTITRUST
AND THE
HEALTH CARE PROVIDER

Martin J. Thompson, J.D.

Memel, Jacobs, Pierno & Gersh

Aspen Systems Corporation
Germantown, Maryland
London, England
1979

Library of Congress Cataloging in Publication Data

Thompson, Martin J.
Antitrust and the health care provider.

Includes index.
1. Health facilities—Law and legislation—United States. 2.
Medical care—Law and legislation—United States. 3. Insurance,
Health—United States. 4. Antitrust law—United States. I. Title.
KF3825.T48   344' .73'03211   79-9371
ISBN 0-89443-159-5

Library of Congress Catalog Card Number: 79-9371
ISBN: 0-89443-159-5

Printed in the United States of America

1 2 3 4 5

To Barbara, my wife

Table of Contents

Preface

A variety of the facets of antitrust law that have proved to be of concern to health care providers is explored in this text. It is hoped that the information will be valuable to lawyers as well as nonlawyers. The footnotes may not interest nonlawyers, but are provided for research assistance and to add certain tangential information. Those interested only in individual chapters should find it unnecessary to read preceding chapters, with the exception of the Introduction, which is recommended as a starting point for those with little or no background in antitrust law.

Martin J. Thompson
October 1979

Acknowledgments

I wish to express my gratitude to my associates—Peter Rich, Hilary Cohen, Jessica Darraby, Cary Davidson, Frank Gruber, and Steven Maler—for their valuable assistance in the preparation of this work.

Chapter 1

Introduction: An Overview of the Antitrust Laws

For most of the years after the first federal antitrust statutes were adopted, those who enforced these laws and those who provided health care services in this country rather pervasively ignored each other. Were it not for disputes created by the early introduction of alternatives to the fee-for-service method of providing care,[1] health care providers might have escaped the attention of enforcers for the first three-quarters of a century after the adoption of the antitrust laws.

The quiet of earlier years, however, has been supplanted recently with a relative frenzy of activity, during which antitrust issues have been posed to providers on an almost continuous basis. The awakening of the antitrust enforcers to the significance of the health care sector of the economy has occurred, perhaps more than coincidentally, with the evolution of the health care industry from its previous and so-called "cottage industry" status to a more modern, sophisticated, and business-like industry; with the introduction of government regulatory programs, originally to stimulate the growth of institutional providers and more recently to restrict the growth of those same institutions; with the pursuit of numerous political positions relating both to expanding the scope of government subsidies for the purchase of health care services and to restricting cost increases in the industry, and the consequent high visibility of the economics of this industry; and with the evolution of the antitrust laws toward new applications in all professions.

The new focus of governmental antitrust enforcers on the health care sector, as well as on other professions and consumer-oriented industries,[2] has not been alone in creating legal disputes for providers. There has been a concurrent increase in efforts by private parties to use antitrust statutes to remedy private disputes. An entirely new and often vague maze of disputes and tensions also has developed between the generally anticompetitive health planning efforts of governmental health planners and providers who, willingly or not, must operate

1

under the health planning processes and the increasing zeal of those who would and do enforce the competition policy represented by the antitrust laws.[3]

Political and legal developments occur constantly in this area, and any particular rule of law may be changed in a moment by legislative or judicial action (and efforts are under way to cause such action to result in new and presumably better rules). Therefore, an understanding of the general and historical applications of antitrust principles and laws, together with consideration of actual attempts to apply these laws in the health care sector, can help providers to monitor and shape their own conduct and that of others upon whom they depend, in order to minimize unnecessary liabilities and recognize redressable grievances. Consequently, this work presents an overview of the pertinent antitrust rules as created by Congress and interpreted by the courts and actual and potential applications of these rules in the health care sector.

STATUTORY OVERVIEW

Compared to the myriad of long and complex statutes and regulations directed specifically at the health care sector, which often seem to be adopted, amended, and replaced on an almost daily basis, the antitrust statutes are few in number, simple in nature, and enjoy an almost unnatural longevity.

The first federal antitrust statute, known as the Sherman Act,[4] was adopted in 1890 and represented the culmination of decades of effort to preclude the formation of monopolies and prevent the abuses of economic power that many had suffered at the hands of the railroads, the Standard Oil Trust, and other economic giants.[5] Although the social background and parts of the legislative history of the Sherman Act sometimes have been taken to indicate a narrow focus upon dealing with the relatively limited number of monopolies and economic abusers of that period, the language of the act and the probable rationale for its existence neither require nor suggest such a narrow scope.[6]

The substantive language of the Sherman Act is contained primarily in the first two sections and has remained essentially unchanged since its adoption in 1890. Section 1[7] provides, in pertinent part, that:

> Every contract, combination in the form of trust or otherwise, or conspiracy, in restraint of trade or commerce among the several States, or with foreign nations, is declared to be illegal.

Certain features of Section 1 deserve special mention. First, the language is noteworthy for its breadth. If particular industries or types of trade were in the minds of members of Congress, these concerns did not reach the point of codification. The act does not distinguish between industries that deal in products and those concerned with services. In fact, the breadth of the language has been said to give the act a desirable type of constitutional sweep, enabling the courts to adapt it to new trades and arrangements as they become troublesome in the economy.[8]

Second, since Section 1 applies only to contracts, combinations, and conspiracies, it necessarily involves only the joint conduct of multiple persons or, more precisely, multiple legal entities (such as separate corporations, other types of businesses, individuals, or combinations of those entities). A single trader, acting individually, cannot violate Section 1 of the Sherman Act, although some courts' constructions of the nature of a conspiracy or combination at times may create the impression that exceedingly little agreement is required to be determined to constitute joint action.

Third, the language of Section 1 could be taken to defeat the legality of virtually any contract or agreement, even those necessary for conducting simple business transactions. For a contract to be of value to a business person, it must be, to some extent, "in restraint of trade." A person who contracts to sell an item to a particular buyer has restricted that individual's ability to sell that item to a competitor of the purchaser. An employee who contracts to provide services to a particular employer similarly restricts the ability to provide those same services to a competitor of the employer.

The courts that were called upon to interpret and apply Section 1 of the Sherman Act soon noted that the common law prohibitions against restraints of trade (*i.e.*, rules developed from English common law and applied primarily by state courts before the Sherman Act was adopted) had not been intended to prohibit restraints necessary for the transaction of business, and the act similarly should not be interpreted to inhibit such conduct. Consequently, the courts have determined that the act was intended to apply only to "unreasonable" restraints of trade.

The case generally credited with first articulating the standard of reasonableness, or "rule of reason," in determining the legality of particular trade restraints is the Supreme Court's 1911 opinion on the conduct of the Standard Oil Trust.[9] The court presented a relatively detailed consideration of the legislative debates that had preceded the adoption of the Sherman Act, concluding that the main cause leading to the act was the economic condition of the times:

> . . . the vast accumulation of wealth in the hands of corporations and individuals, the enormous development of corporate organization, the facility for combination which such organizations afforded, the fact that the facility was being used, and that combinations known as trusts were being multiplied, and the widespread impression that their power had been and would be exerted to oppress individuals and injure the public generally.[10]

Considering the legal and economic history of this country, the Supreme Court expressed the policy rationale and explanation for Section 1 of the Sherman Act with the following conclusion:

> In view of the common law and the law in this country as to restraint of trade, which we have reviewed, and the illuminating effect which that history must have under the rule to which we have referred, we think it results:
>
> a. That the context manifests that the statute was drawn in the light of the existing practical conception of the law of restraint of trade, because it groups as within that class, not only contracts which were in restraint of trade in the subjective sense, but all contracts or acts which theoretically were attempts to monopolize, yet which in practice had come to be considered as in restraint of trade in a broad sense.
>
> b. That in view of the many new forms of contracts and combinations which were being evolved from existing economic conditions, it was deemed essential by an all-embracing enumeration to make sure that no form of contract or combination by which an undue restraint of interstate or foreign commerce was brought about could save such restraint from condemnation. The statute under this view evidenced the intent not to restrain the right to make and enforce contracts, whether resulting from combinations or otherwise, which did not unduly restrain interstate or foreign commerce, but to protect that commerce from being restrained by methods, whether old or new, which would constitute an interference,—that is, an undue restraint.[11]

The court specifically disapproved the government's contention that the act should be interpreted to disallow every restraint of trade, explaining that the failure to define "restraint of trade" indicated that the law was expressly designed to allow broad application and:

> . . . to leave it to be determined by the light of reason, guided by the principles of law and the duty to apply and enforce the public policy embodied in the statute, in every given case whether any particular act or contract was within the contemplation of the statute.[12]

The "rule of reason" test articulated by the Supreme Court in 1911 quite clearly is a vague approach to the resolution of lawsuits and allows tremendous room for the development of more specific guidelines for courts and litigants to follow in applying Section 1. In 1918 the Supreme Court again addressed the reasonableness of an alleged restraint of trade and issued what still is considered the classic statement of guidelines for applying the rule of reason:

The true test of legality is whether the restraint imposed is such as merely regulates and perhaps thereby promotes competition or whether it is such as may suppress or even destroy competition. To determine that question the court must ordinarily consider the facts peculiar to the business to which the restraint is applied; its condition before and after the restraint was imposed; the nature of the restraint and its effect, actual or probable. The history of the restraint, the evil believed to exist, the reason for adopting the particular remedy, the purpose or end sought to be attained, are all relevant facts. This is not because a good intention will save an otherwise objectionable regulation or the reverse; but because knowledge of intent may help the court to interpret facts and to predict consequences.[13]

To establish that a particular agreement or trade practice is unreasonable and a violation of Section 1 involves extensive factual proofs, perhaps addressing all of the factors discussed by the Supreme Court, and almost certainly requiring the use of economists and complex economic analysis of the industry and restraints in question. Perhaps predictably, then, the courts at times have become uncomfortable with this cumbersome process and have developed simpler rules that may be applied in particular circumstances. In cases involving different types of trade restraints, the courts have determined that where a particular type of restraint is demonstrated, the need for supporting economic and historical analysis may be eliminated. In essence, the courts have held that certain restraints are inherently so unreasonable that the mere fact that the restraint exists is sufficient to demonstrate its illegality. These restraints therefore are determined to be unreasonable and illegal in and of themselves or, as more popularly stated, are *per se* unreasonable and illegal.

In 1958, the Supreme Court offered an explanation and summary of the offenses that by then had been determined to be unreasonable *per se:*

However, there are certain agreements or practices which because of their pernicious effect on competition and lack of any redeeming virtue are conclusively presumed to be unreasonable and therefore illegal without elaborate inquiry as to the precise harm they have caused or the business excuse for their use. This principle of *per se* unreasonableness not only makes the type of restraints which are proscribed by the Sherman Act more certain to the benefit of everyone concerned, but it also avoids the necessity for an incredibly complicated and prolonged economic investigation into the entire history of the industry involved, as well as related industries, in an effort to determine at large whether a particular restraint has been unreasonable—an inquiry so often wholly fruitless when undertaken. Among the practices which the courts have heretofore deemed to be unlawful in and of themselves

are price fixing, division of markets, group boycotts, and tying arrangements, ...[14]

The variety of agreements and practices that may be determined under given
circumstances to constitute unreasonable and therefore illegal restraints of trade
is virtually unlimited and consequently not amenable to consideration on a prac-
tice-by-practice basis. However, the types of restraints that the Supreme Court
deemed to be unlawful *per se,* as noted, do merit some explanation and consideration on an individual basis.

Price Fixing

Price fixing, a *per se* violation of the Sherman Act, can refer to a number of
practices. In the classic sense, it generally refers to an agreement among competitors establishing a common price, or system for setting the prices, of their
products. The term also can encompass agreements among competitors relating
to the prices they will pay for products that they all must purchase, agreements
among competitors on the manner in which they will or will not bid for various
contractual rights, and restrictions by the seller of a product on the price at which
the purchaser may resell that product. Primarily because price competition generally is perceived to be the very foundation of a competitive economic system,
each form of price fixing described has been regarded consistently as a *per se*
antitrust violation, illegal in itself.[15]

In fact, the Supreme Court has explained that any combination that tampers
with the price structure or pricing mechanism is engaged in an unlawful activity,
even absent an actual agreement on particular prices.[16] The fact that the combination may only effectuate an agreement to fix prices at the going market rate,
or that a particular agreement may have the effect of reducing rather than raising
prices, will not save the combination or agreement from illegality.[17]

Although the applications of these general rules are discussed in more detail
in subsequent chapters, the most popular application of the antiprice-fixing rules
in the health care industry probably has involved physicians' relative value
schedules, whereby various medical associations have published lists of charges
for different types of procedures. The schedules generally did not require adherence by physicians and did not actually establish a price for any particular procedure. However, the practice could tend to influence the pricing mechanism
and the actual cost of services to the extent that physicians conformed to the
relative charges suggested by the schedules. Consequently, in all reported instances in which the schedules have been challenged, the physicians' associations involved have consented to terminate the practice.

Other troublesome areas involving pricing of health care services have included association activities in disseminating information on past prices and

costs of various products and services—information that might have been abused by the group's members as a means of arriving at informal mechanisms for stabilizing prices. Similarly, the dissemination of wage scales, especially when coupled with forecasts of wages and suggestions to conform to those forecasts, may lead to agreements influencing salaries paid to employees of providers— another form of price fixing.

Division of Markets

The *per se* violation of dividing markets refers to agreements among competitors who determine to allocate certain markets to certain of the participants, thereby reducing or eliminating competition among them in a market. The Supreme Court described this type of market allocation, and the violation it constitutes, in a 1972 opinion:

> One of the classic examples of a *per se* violation of §1 is an agreement between competitors at the same level of the market structure to allocate territories in order to minimize competition. Such concerted action is usually termed a "horizontal" restraint, in contradistinction to combinations of persons at different levels of the market structure, *e.g.*, manufacturers and distributors, which are termed "vertical" restraints. This Court has reiterated time and time again that "horizontal territorial limitations . . . are naked restraints of trade with no purpose except the stifling of competition." . . . Such limitations are *per se* violations of the Sherman Act.[18]

One of the more interesting applications of the rule disallowing the division of markets among competitors or potential competitors arises in the health planning context. Quite simply, one of the major thrusts of many health planning agencies is to allocate markets among hospitals in order to eliminate competition among various services and thereby end duplication of efforts in an attempt to reduce the amount of capital expended in providing these services. Conversely, however, this activity involves the creation of local monopolies or at least the reduction of competition among these institutional providers. Under the standards cited above, these activities ordinarily would be presumed to be *per se* violations of Section 1 of the Sherman Act. Under particular circumstances, however, various immunities may be available to protect this health planning conduct. These potential immunities are discussed in Chapter 3.

Group Boycotts

Although a group boycott is considered a *per se* violation of Section 1, attaching the label "group boycott" to particular conduct often is more the result of a conclusion that the activity is illegal than it is a functional description of that activity. In essence, a group boycott is a form of concerted refusal to deal in which one group of persons or legal entities has chosen jointly not to deal in business with some other person or group. However, whether a concerted refusal to deal actually amounts to a *per se* illegal group boycott often is a more difficult question than it might first appear to be.

The classic case on the *per se* illegality rule for group boycotts is the Supreme Court's 1959 decision in *Klor's, Inc. v. Broadway-Hale Stores, Inc.*,[19] where the court explained that:

> Group boycotts, or concerted refusals by traders to deal with other traders, have long been held to be in the forbidden category [*i.e.*, *per se* violations]. They have not been saved by allegations that they were reasonable in the specific circumstances, nor by a failure to show that they "fixed or regulated prices, parcelled out or limited production, or brought about a deterioration in quality." . . . Even when they operated to lower prices or temporarily to stimulate competition they were banned.[20]

Subsequent courts have explained, however, that the "group boycott" label for particular conduct should be restricted to relatively narrow practices. For example, one court ruled in 1978 that the National Football League player draft was not a "group boycott" deserving of *per se* treatment under the Sherman Act. The court stated that:

> The "group boycott" designation, we believe, is properly restricted to concerted attempts by competitors to exclude horizontal competitors; it should not be applied, and has never been applied by the Supreme Court, to concerted refusals that are not designed to drive out competitors but to achieve some other goal.
>
> . . . The courts have consistently refused to invoke the boycott *per se* rule where, given the peculiar characteristics of an industry, the need for cooperation among participants necessitated some type of concerted refusal to deal, or where the concerted activity manifested no purpose to exclude and in fact worked no exclusion of competitors.[21]

The boycott, or concerted refusal to deal, historically has been a particularly fruitful area for the application of antitrust principles in the health care industry. A disproportionately large number of the disputes have concerned the introduction of nonphysician and nonfee-for-service methods of providing health care services, together with perceptions by those introducing the new methods that various groups in the health care establishment might have used their positions to inhibit the growth of these alternative methods through conduct in the nature of boycotts, as well as other types of actions.

In 1943, in the Supreme Court's first significant consideration of restraints of trade in the health care industry, for example,[22] the government contended that the American Medical Association and the Medical Society of the District of Columbia, together with various members of those associations, had conspired to inhibit or prevent the operation of a prepaid health plan. The conspiracy was alleged to have included efforts by physician members of the associations to cause other physicians not to deal with the prepaid plan and threats to expel from the association physicians who did deal with the plan. Although the court did not refer to this as a "boycott," the conduct in question clearly could be so characterized. In subsequent years, health maintenance organizations have raised contentions of boycotts by various associations and other entities with which they must deal. Similarly, governmental enforcers fear that established medical associations and other groups will use their positions to effectively boycott the pursuit of low cost, predominantly nonphysician forms of care, such as nurse practitioners and the clinics they may operate with only minimal physician assistance.[23]

Other refusals to deal by organized associations have raised numerous boycott questions, as associations frequently establish membership requirements that exclude certain would-be members, perhaps to the economic disadvantage of the excluded persons (who may be actual or potential competitors of members). Moreover, medical staffs that act to exclude some applicant physicians may well encounter allegations of anticompetitive boycotts, as the excluded physicians are rendered unable to compete in a particular hospital and perhaps in an entire locality. These and other boycott issues are discussed in Chapter 5 on association activities and Chapter 6 on medical staff privileges.

It is important to note, however, that the rules on group boycotts and other concerted refusals to deal apply only to joint conduct. An individual decision to refuse to do business with someone is not illegal unless it amounts to monopolizing. The Supreme Court has explained:

> In the absence of any purpose to create or maintain a monopoly the [Sherman] act does not restrict the long recognized right of trader or manufacturer engaged in an entirely private business, freely to exercise his own independent discretion as to parties with whom he will deal; . . .[24]

Tying Arrangements

A tying arrangement is a situation in which a party agrees to sell a certain product or service only on the condition that the buyer also purchases a different product or service, or at least agrees not to purchase that product or service from another supplier. The first product is referred to as the "tying product" and the second as the "tied product." Where these arrangements involve commodities rather than services, they generally are attacked under the more specific language of the Clayton Act (see page twelve). However, where services are involved in the tying arrangement, the arrangement may become a *per se* violation of Section 1 of the Sherman Act.

Although the Supreme Court has called tying arrangements *per se* violations of the Sherman Act, the proof of the tying arrangement itself is not adequate to demonstrate the violation of the act. The entirety of the test of legality described by the Supreme Court essentially is as follows:

1. The arrangement must involve two separate products or services, as opposed to a single product or service with definable but essentially inseparable subparts.
2. The seller must enjoy sufficient economic power with respect to the tying product to appreciably restrain free competition in the market for the tied product.
3. A not insubstantial amount of interstate commerce must be affected by the arrangement.[25]

Potential applications of this doctrine in the health care industry include the activities of association and shared service organizations that may well tie the providing of one service to an agreement to participate similarly in other services. For example, if a shared service organization that operates as a group buying unit will not allow members to participate in the buying function for one product unless those members also purchase other products through the group arrangement, then tying issues are raised. Similarly, if a hospital will not allow physicians to use hospital beds unless they also agree to use the hospital laboratory service, tying issues also may be raised. The resolution of these issues will depend upon the determination of each of the factors listed above, as well as the potential reliance upon defenses such as the necessity for providing assurances of quality in medical care in order to avoid hospital liability in connection with physician malpractice actions.

SHERMAN ACT—SECTION 2

Section 2 of the Sherman Act is directed explicitly at prohibiting monopolizing, whether by an individual or a group. The relevant portion of this section provides:

> Every person who shall monopolize, or attempt to monopolize, or combine or conspire with any other person or persons, to monopolize

any part of the trade or commerce among the several States, or with foreign nations, shall be deemed guilty of a felony . . .[26]

The determination of illegal monopolization depends upon three elements: (1) the defendant's possession of monopoly power within a relevant market; (2) the defendant's acquisition or maintenance of this power by exclusionary or anticompetitive means or the use of the power for exclusionary or anticompetitive purposes; and (3) injury to the plaintiff as a result of the monopoly power and exclusionary or anticompetitive conduct.[27] The first question, therefore, is what constitutes monopoly power? While the valid answer is that monopoly power is the power to raise prices or exclude competitors, this may prove hard to work with in evaluating practical situations.

In 1945, the Court of Appeals for the Second Circuit was presented with a situation in which the market share of a company charged with monopolization could be measured in any of three different ways.[28] Depending upon the manner of measurement, the defendant company enjoyed either 33, 64, or 90 percent of the American aluminum market. The court determined that in the circumstances of that case, 90 percent would constitute a monopoly, 33 percent would not, and 64 percent was considered doubtful. While numerous other examples of market shares held to establish the existence of a monopoly could be considered,[29] each situation depends upon the circumstances of the individual market, in order to determine whether the market share and the power of the company enables that company unilaterally to raise prices or exclude competitors.

The second element, that of the use of anticompetitive or exclusionary tactics in connection with the acquisition or maintenance of the monopoly power, relates back to the language of the statute. It is important that the statute does not purport to state that holding a monopoly is illegal in itself. Rather, the conduct of monopolizing is what is illegal. Consequently, where the acquisition of monopoly power is the result of honest industrial effort or superior business acumen, or where the monopoly power is thrust upon a defendant through the circumstances of the situation, monopolization has not necessarily occurred. Monopolization has occurred only where monopoly power is acquired or maintained through means that are not economically inevitable or honestly calculated only to serve the interests of consumers rather than to hinder the efforts of competitors.

Applying the concept of monopolization and the related concepts of attempt to monopolize and conspiracy to monopolize in the health care industry raises particular difficulties. The regulatory processes that pervade this industry themselves create such significant barriers to entry that the creation or maintenance of monopoly power frequently may be a function of government regulation rather than private monopolization. Furthermore, the measurement of monopoly power is made unusually complex because of the frequent irrelevance of the ordinary issues relating to the ability to raise prices or exclude competitors. However, where monopolization can and does occur in this industry through the conduct of private parties and without the defense of government regulation, then the ordinary rules should apply here as in other industries.

THE CONCEPT OF CONSPIRACY

As both Sections 1 and 2 of the Sherman Act disallow, among other things, a conspiracy to effectuate unlawful restraints of trade or to monopolize, participants in group conduct should be familiar with the nature of "conspiracy" as used in the antitrust laws. Although the essence of a conspiracy is an agreement to reach an unlawful end, or a lawful end through unlawful means, the parties may be found to be coconspirators even though no formal agreement is proved.[30] One federal court in 1978 explained many of the relevant rules on the proof of a conspiracy, stating:

> . . . the formalities of the usual business contract are neither required nor expected. No formal agreement is necessary to constitute an unlawful conspiracy. Often crimes are a matter of inference deduced from the acts of the person accused and done in pursuance of a criminal purpose . . . Tacit understanding created and executed by a long course of conduct is enough to constitute agreement even without personal communication. . . . The form or manner of making the agreement are not crucial . . . The proof, by the nature of the crime, must be circumstantial and therefore inferential to an extent varying with the conditions under which the crime may be committed . . . Once the conspiracy has been established, slight evidence is needed to connect a particular participant . . . Even a single act may be sufficient to draw a defendant within the ambit of a conspiracy where the act is such that one may infer from it an intent to participate in the unlawful enterprise . . . Participation in a criminal conspiracy need not be proved by direct evidence; a common purpose can be inferred from a development and a collocation of circumstances.[31]

Naturally, the possibility that an inference of conspiracy may be drawn from group and association conduct is a particularly troublesome area and is an issue to which all health care providers who engage in group and association activities must be sensitive. These matters are discussed in greater detail in Chapter 5 on group and association activities.

THE CLAYTON ACT

The "constitutional sweep" of the Sherman Act notwithstanding, after 24 years Congress determined that more specificity in the antitrust statutes might be helpful. Consequently, in 1914 the Clayton Act[32] was adopted. The Clayton Act provides new forms of substantive offenses, new standards for demonstrating violations, new methods of enforcement and forms of relief, and new exemptions from antitrust scrutiny. The substantive offenses introduced by the Clayton Act include the following:

Section 3 of the Clayton Act[33] invalidates exclusive dealings and tying arrangements where the effect of that conduct "may be to substantially lessen competition or tend to create a monopoly in any line of commerce." Unlike the Sherman Act, this section covers only conduct involving commodities and does not reach exclusive dealing and tying arrangements that relate to services. Consequently, where services are involved in exclusive dealing or tying arrangements, the more general standards of the Sherman Act must be used. Case law over the years, however, has tended to apply essentially similar tests of illegality to tying and exclusive dealing arrangements, whether the Clayton Act or Sherman Act is applied.[34] Section 3 of the Clayton Act also contains a different jurisdictional standard than that in the Sherman Act, requiring that the challenged conduct be "in commerce" rather than merely "affecting commerce." The significance of this difference is discussed later.

Exclusive dealing arrangements have been of unusual significance in the health care sector and have been the subject of numerous judicial opinions. Although the Clayton Act restricts only arrangements that relate to commodities, an exclusive dealing arrangement involving services may be subject to scrutiny as a contract in restraint of trade under Sherman Act standards. Consequently, an exclusive services contract between a hospital and a professional medical corporation, for the operation of a particular hospital department, might be subject to the Sherman Act if other jurisdictional requirements are met.

While exclusive dealing arrangements never have been subjected to a *per se* type of rule, the courts generally have recognized the economic hardship that may occur where these arrangements preclude competitors from a significant number of sources of supply or of outlets for the purchase of goods or services. Where a market is so affected by exclusive dealing arrangements that competition is substantially foreclosed, the agreements have been scrutinized closely. However, the continuing recognition that some exclusive dealing agreements serve beneficial purposes, such as providing dependable sources of supply where needed, prevents them from being considered *per se* invalid.[35]

Section 7 of the Clayton Act[36] specifically prohibits corporate acquisitions where the effect may be to lessen competition substantially or to tend to create a monopoly. Although this section is considered in detail in Chapter 4 on consolidations and affiliations, it merits attention at this point because it may well be applicable to many multiinstitutional arrangements such as providers' creation of joint venture corporations to eliminate duplicate services as well as to stabilize or better capture markets. As with other areas of tension between antitrust law and health care regulation, where regulatory pressures actually lead to multiin-stitutional arrangements, certain exemptions may be relevant in protecting that conduct from antitrust prosecution.

Section 8 of the Clayton Act[37] specifically disallows certain interlocking di-rectorates and officers; this is discussed in detail in a subsequent chapter. It is of particular importance in the health care industry because of the frequently over-lapping representation of individuals on hospital boards. Because of Section 8, it is entirely possible that well-meaning civic-minded persons who serve on nu-merous local boards may be violating the antitrust laws.

Section 2 of the Clayton Act[38] establishes the illegality of certain price dis-crimination in the sale or purchase of commodities. This section was amended in 1936 by the Robinson-Patman Act and generally is referred to as the Robin-son-Patman Act rather than as a subsection of the Clayton Act. The Robinson-Patman Act is the subject of Chapter 8 and will not be considered in detail here. Generally. this section relates only to transactions in the purchase and sale of commodities of like grade and quality, where the purchases or sales are made at different prices without appropriate justification. The section is the product of depression legislation and has been criticized severely for perceived anticompet-itive effects, as it tends to inhibit some price negotiating that necessarily would lead to favorable treatment for those who negotiate better than others. Neverthe-less, it is a valid and enforceable statute which must be considered when provi-ders purchase or sell commodities within interstate commerce.

THE FEDERAL TRADE COMMISSION ACT

Along with the specificity of the Clayton Act, the year 1914 brought with it the breadth and generality of the substantive offenses encompassed by the Fed-eral Trade Commission Act,[39] as well as the creation of the Federal Trade Com-mission (FTC) that enforces that act. The Federal Trade Commission Act ad-dresses conduct that is anticompetitive or of a deceptive and unfair nature that is beyond the scope of antitrust principles. Section 5 of that act establishes the substantive violations. Although this section is long, the basic operative provi-sion is the first sentence:

> Unfair methods of competition in or affecting commerce, and unfair or
> deceptive acts or practices in or affecting commerce, are declared un-
> lawful.[40]

The act empowers the FTC to enforce this statute, to conduct investigations of possible violations, and to promulgate rules to help provide specificity in pre-venting unfair and deceptive acts and practices. Although the language of Sec-tion 5 of the FTC act is itself so broad and general that, on its face, it offers little assistance in the interpretation of this statute, the courts have explained that the act encompasses the same sort of conduct as would violate the Sherman Act and also allows the FTC to prohibit unfair acts even where such acts are beyond the scope of the Sherman Act.[41] Where particular conduct might be "unfair" and have the effect of restraining or foreclosing competition through effects that either affect free competition adversely or create an incipient menace to the existence of free competition, then the FTC act may be violated.[42]

The FTC's investigative powers are established in Section 6 of its act,[43] which confers upon the Commission the general power to gather and compile information concerning, and to investigate, businesses and conduct that affect commerce.

In spite of the tremendous breadth and generality of the FTC act, its operation is subject to an exception that is extremely pertinent in the health care industry. In this respect, Section 4[44] provides definitions to be used in interpreting the substantive provisions. The definition of "corporation," while including any associations whether incorporated or not, specifically excludes entities that are not organized for the profit of that business or the profit of the members of that business or association. Consequently, the Commission does not enjoy enforcement jurisdiction over nonprofit health care providers. However, it does have such jurisdiction over nonprofit associations organized for the profit of their members, such as the American Medical Association and other professional societies. This explicit jurisdictional limitation does not exempt nonprofit organizations from requirements to comply with investigative demands of the Commission, as these demands may be used toward establishing violations committed by other, profit-making, enterprises.[45]

The Federal Trade Commission has been particularly active in investigating and prosecuting health care providers for various alleged unfair trade practices. In fact, the chairman has commented specifically upon the commission's new focus on the health care industry as well as other consumer-oriented industries,[46] and investigations have been pursued relating to: physician dominance of Blue Shield programs, the use of relative value schedules by medical associations, the possibility that physicians may use board certification as an excuse to extend their own monopoly power, conduct calculated to inhibit the growth of health maintenance organizations, the removal of restraints on advertising, potential anticompetitive practices in medical school accreditation, and other areas.

JURISDICTIONAL CONSIDERATIONS

The limitation of the Sherman Act, to the effect that it applies only to restraints of "trade or commerce among the several states, or with foreign nations," generally has been interpreted to extend the act's reach to any conduct that has a substantial effect on interstate commerce.[47] The question of the impact of the activities of health care providers upon interstate commerce, however, has been the subject of major dispute when prosecutors have attempted to apply the Sherman Act to the health care industry.

Although some observers apparently concluded originally that health care providers were virtually incapable of creating a substantial impact upon interstate commerce, the Supreme Court in a 1976 opinion explained just how an alleged conspiracy to prevent the construction of a new hospital could create an impact on interstate commerce sufficient to confer jurisdiction under the Sherman Act. In *Hospital Building Company v. Trustees of Rex Hospital*,[48] the Court held that the construction of the hospital in issue would involve purchases of supplies that traveled through interstate commerce, as well as arrangements for financing from out-of-state lenders, and consequently, a conspiracy that prevented the construction of the hospital would impact upon this interstate commerce. Subsequently, courts have found much smaller restraints of trade in the health care industry to offer the potential impact upon interstate commerce necessary to confer Sherman Act jurisdiction. For example, in a 1977 case a federal trial court ruled that the exclusion from a hospital of a single physician could impact substantially upon interstate commerce if that physician's patients included persons who received reimbursement through federal subsidy programs such as Medicare. The inability of this physician to conduct his practice thus would restrict the flow of these Medicare funds through interstate commerce, the court said, and thereby impact upon that interstate commerce sufficiently to confer Sherman Act jurisdiction.[49]

Where a contract, combination, or conspiracy restrains trade or commerce in the District of Columbia or in any territory of the United States, it can be actionable without a showing of impact upon interstate commerce, under Section 3 of the Sherman Act. This section essentially repeats the operative language of Section 1, with application only to the District of Columbia and the territories, and requires only a showing that trade has been restrained in one of those areas, or between one of those areas and any state, or between one of those areas and foreign nations. Consequently, where physicians were accused of restraining commerce in health care services in the District of Columbia, the conduct was actionable under Section 3 without any demonstration of impact upon interstate commerce.[50]

The Federal Trade Commission Act, while using somewhat different language, applies essentially the same interstate commerce requirement as does the Sherman Act. Thus, although the Federal Trade Commission Act refers specifically to "in or affecting commerce," the circumstances under which a substantial impact upon interstate commerce confers Sherman Act jurisdiction should apply equally to Section 5 of the Federal Trade Commission Act.

The Clayton Act, unlike the Sherman and Federal Trade Commission Acts, however, does not reach all persons or all conduct that merely impact upon interstate commerce. The specific provisions of Section 2 (price discrimination),

Section 3 (tying and exclusive dealing), Section 7 (corporate acquisitions), and Section 8 (interlocking directorates) refer to corporations and persons "engaged in commerce" rather than conduct that merely affects commerce. The distinction between a business that merely affects commerce and one engaged in commerce is that a provider that engages in strictly local purchases and sales and renders services only on a local (intrastate) basis nevertheless may impact upon commerce, while to be "engaged in commerce," that provider actually must make purchases or sales across state lines. For example, a hospital may be engaged in interstate commerce if it purchases drugs directly from out-of-state suppliers.

THE IMPORTANCE OF STATE ANTITRUST STATUTES

Because of the occasional difficulty of demonstrating the requisite effect upon interstate commerce, or perhaps showing that the defendant is engaged in commerce, a substantial number of restraint of trade cases in the health care industry have been pursued in state courts, either under state statutes or as common law causes of action. All states have laws prohibiting various restraints of trade. Most of these state laws, to a greater or lesser extent, conform to the standards and policies established by the Sherman Act. Many of these state statutes are even referred to as "little Sherman Acts." Consequently, where interstate commerce may present a problem to a plaintiff in an antitrust action, the availability of state law should not be overlooked.

Because state laws may be interpreted somewhat differently from the Sherman Act and other federal antitrust statutes, it is possible that the scope of the laws may be somewhat different from that indicated by the prevailing interpretation of the Sherman Act. For example, some state laws may not be interpreted to reach the professions, such as the practice of medicine, whereas the Sherman Act is interpreted on a broader basis.[51]

Even beyond state antitrust statutes is the potential application of common law—uncodified rules prohibiting unreasonable restraints of trade. At least one state court has determined that its own state antitrust laws, as well as the Sherman Act, simply apply common law standards and therefore, even if the state statutes and the Sherman Act might not apply to particular conduct because of some statutory restriction, a similar rule of reason standard may be applied under common law principles.[52]

EXEMPTIONS AND EXCLUSIONS

Exemptions and exclusions that may protect health care providers from antitrust scrutiny are found in three basic sources: (1) those created specifically by antitrust statutes, (2) those created by health care statutes, (3) those created by the courts in interpreting and applying combinations of antitrust and health care laws.

Exemptions created by antitrust statutes that may be relevant to health care providers are as follows:

Section 6 of the Clayton Act[53] creates an exemption for labor and agricultural organizations set up for purposes of mutual help and not conducted for profit. Under this section, together with certain labor-oriented statutes, labor unions may pursue activities that otherwise would violate the antitrust laws. For example, a labor strike could well constitute a group boycott in violation of the Sherman Act were it not for the exemption created by Section 6 of the Clayton Act.

At least one attempt has been made to amend Section 6 of the Clayton Act to similarly exempt associations of health professions personnel from antitrust scrutiny. This attempt, however, did not pass Congress.[54]

Section 2c of the Clayton Act[55]—part of the Robinson-Patman Act—provides an exemption from the rule against price discrimination for purchases of supplies by nonprofit hospitals and other charitable institutions where the supplies are bought for the institution's own use. This exemption is discussed in detail in Chapter 8 on price discrimination.

As previously noted, Section 4 of the Federal Trade Commission Act excludes nonprofit institutions that are not operated for the profit of their members from the FTC's enforcement jurisdiction.

The insurance business is exempted specifically from the antitrust laws to the extent that it is regulated by state law. This statutory exemption, however, does not exempt boycott activities. The exemption is particularly important to health care providers, as they are forced to deal so closely with insurers for purposes of reimbursement, and because in these dealings providers either may encounter redressable grievances by the insurance companies or may be accused of coconspiring with insurance companies in various illegal activities. The insurance exemption from the antitrust laws is discussed in Chapter 7 on relations with insurers.

The creation of specific antitrust exemptions through health-related statutes has been of recent concern and discussion and undoubtedly will see significant future developments. At present, however, the statutory exemptions are narrow in nature and probably of relatively little value in and of themselves.

For example, Section 1512(b)(4) of Public Law 93-641 (the National Health Planning and Resources Development Act of 1974) provides a limited immunity for individuals acting as members or employees of health systems agencies. The immunity is specifically limited, however, to conduct in which the individual ". . . has acted within the scope of such duty, function, or activity, has exercised due care, and has acted, with respect to that performance, without malice toward any person affected by it." Consequently, where a member or employee of a Health Systems Agency has acted beyond the scope of the appropriate duties, functions, or activities of that agency (presumably no matter how ill-defined the scope of those activities may be), the immunity may be lost.

Similarly, the law involving Professional Standards Review Organizations (PSROs) provides a limited immunity for the conduct of members and employees of these groups. This immunity also is limited, however, to conduct in the performance of a duty, function, or activity authorized or required of PSROs or Statewide Professional Standards Review councils. Consequently, if the conduct is outside of the scope of required or authorized activities, no immunity is provided.[56]

The health care exemptions described above are limited to creating immunities for members and employees of certain public agencies and do not confer immunity upon providers acting under the direction of, or in concert with, those public agencies. Moreover, these statutes do not even immunize the members and employees of the agencies to the extent that their conduct later is determined to have been outside of the scope of the proper functions of the agencies. The most promising exemptions and immunities available now to health care providers are those created by judicial interpretations and applications of the antitrust laws as necessary to resolve conflicts between antitrust statutes and other regulatory statutes, as well as to resolve conflicts between antitrust policy and certain Constitutional guarantees.

The Supreme Court has held that the First Amendment protects even joint and concerted efforts, including those for specifically anticompetitive purposes, to influence the political processes of the legislatures or legislative-type bodies. Similarly, a somewhat narrower First Amendment immunity is available for joint efforts to influence governmental adjudicatory bodies, such as administrative tribunals and courts. Consequently, where health care providers join together in the effort to influence these types of governmental agencies, even for purposes of putting rivals out of business or with other anticompetitive motives and effects, the conduct may be immunized from antitrust attack. This immunity is discussed in Chapter 5 on efforts to influence governmental processes.

The antitrust laws are deemed to be repealed by implication to the minimum extent necessary to allow other federal regulatory statutes to operate. In addition, the laws have been determined to be inapplicable to the conduct of state officers in pursuit of valid state regulatory schemes and to the conduct of private parties under the compulsion of a valid state regulatory scheme. These "implied repeal" and "state action" exemptions are discussed in Chapter 3.

It was believed at one time that the Sherman Act and other federal antitrust laws did not apply to the conduct of members of the learned professions, such as physicians and attorneys. The Supreme Court, however, terminated any such beliefs with its opinion in a 1975 case titled *Goldfarb v. Virginia State Bar*.[57] In that case, the Supreme Court clearly stated that there simply was no exemption from the antitrust laws for those engaged in the learned professions. The court has continued to recognize, however, that the antitrust laws may apply to learned professions in a somewhat different manner from the way they are applied to other forms of business.[58] Exactly how differently the law will be applied to the learned professions is yet to be determined.

ENFORCEMENT AND PENALTY CONSIDERATIONS

The penalties for violation of the antitrust laws can be severe. Violations of the Sherman Act can lead to both criminal and civil prosecutions, while most violations of the Clayton Act (other than certain portions of the Robinson-Patman Act) can result in civil prosecutions only.

Enforcement of the antitrust laws can be pursued by the Antitrust Division of the Department of Justice, in certain instances by the Federal Trade Commission, by state attorneys general, and, where authority is delegated, by certain local government attorneys, as well as by private parties seeking damages. Certain particularly relevant enforcement considerations include the following:

Sections 1 and 2 of the Sherman Act specifically make violation of that statute a potential felony, providing for both monetary fines and jail sentences.

Section 4 of the Clayton Act creates a cause of action on behalf of any person injured in his business or property by reason of an antitrust violation for three times the actual damages, together with reasonable attorneys' fees.

Enforcement of the antitrust laws also can include equitable relief, such as injunctions, monitoring of businesses found to be violators, and, in some instances, dissolution of illegal enterprises.

Although the penalties for violation of the antitrust laws may be severe, there are certain limitations on the classes of individuals who may bring private actions to enforce these laws. In particular, the Supreme Court held in 1977 that only the direct purchaser of a product (or presumably a service) that had suffered inflated charges due to antitrust violations could bring suit for those violations. The court added that subsequent purchasers—those who paid inflated prices later in the chain of distribution but who did not deal directly with the alleged antitrust violator—could not bring suit against the alleged violation.[59] This decision somewhat restricted the scope of potential plaintiffs in antitrust actions and has been the subject of substantial criticism. A bill introduced in the United States Senate early in 1979 would permit actions against alleged antitrust violations to be brought by those who did not deal directly with the alleged violator but who nevertheless paid inflated charges because of the alleged violation.[60]

TRENDS AND DEVELOPMENTS

The extent to which the Sherman Act has succeeded in its role as a "comprehensive charter of economic liberty aimed at preserving free and unfettered competition as the rule of trade''[61] has been questioned in recent years. On January 22, 1979, a special commission appointed by the President to review the antitrust laws and procedures issued a report on the history and effectiveness of the laws and recommended modifications. Of particular interest to health care providers should be the consideration of regulated industries. The commission recommended an increased emphasis on reliance on competition rather than regulation to solve the problems of regulated industries.

While the commission did not refer directly to the health care industry, it did call for elimination of exemptions and regulatory schemes not currently justified, and an examination of antitrust immunities to determine which were necessary. The commission also urged that competition be a principal consideration in regulatory agency decision making. While changes in the antitrust laws generally come slowly, it was anticipated that the recommended modifications would be presented to Congress for consideration.

In general, the trend of the times could be summarized as an increasing effort by health planners and health care regulators to remove many barriers to the elimination of competition among providers through the health planning process, and the concurrent emphasis by antitrust enforcers to eliminate barriers to competition created by the regulatory process. It probably is too early to predict a winner from these occasionally contradictory movements.

NOTES

1. The dispute addressed by the Supreme Court in *American Medical Ass'n v. United States,* 317 U.S. 519, 63 S.Ct. 326 (1943), is the first major instance of applying antitrust principles to health providers. Even after this early case, little activity occurred within the area for close to 30 years.

2. *See,* for example, the remarks of Michael Pertschuk, chairman of the Federal Trade Commission, reprinted in Antitrust & Trade Reg. Rep. (BNA) No. 840, November 24, 1977.

3. *Note,* for example, the plight of the Central Virginia Health Systems Agency, which developed an ambitious health systems plan and annual implementation plan, only to be informed that its program would violate the antitrust laws.

4. 15 U.S.C.

5. For an extensive discussion of the historical background of the Sherman Act, *see* Letwin, "CONGRESS AND THE SHERMAN ANTITRUST LAW: 1887–1890," 23 U.Chi. L. Rev. 221 (1956).

6. The legislative history of the Sherman Act, including extensive discussion of legislative debates and amendments to the act, is considered in detail in Volumes 2 and 3 of Von Kalinowski, *Antitrust.*

7. 15 U.S.C. § 1.

8. *See, e.g., Appalachian Coals, Inc. v. United States,* 228 U.S. 344, 53 S.Ct. 471 (1933).

9. *Standard Oil Co. v. United States,* 221 U.S. 1, 31 S.Ct. 502 (1911).

10. *Id.,* at 50, 31 S.Ct. 512.

11. *Id.,* at 59–60, 31 S.Ct. 515.

12. *Id.,* at 63–64, 31 S.Ct. 517.

13. *Board of Trade of City of Chicago v. United States,* 246 U.S. 231, 238, 38 S.Ct. 242, 244 (1918).

14. *Northern Pacific Ry. Co. v. United States*, 356 U.S. 1, 5, 78 S.Ct. 514, 518 (1958).

15. *Cf., United States v. Socony-Vacuum Oil Co., Inc.*, 310 U.S. 150, 60 S.Ct. 811 (1940).

16. *Id.*

17. *Id.*

18. *United States v. Topco Associates, Inc.*, 405 U.S. 596, 608, 92 S.Ct. 1126, 1133–1134 (1972).

19. 359 U.S. 207, 79 S.Ct. 705 (1959).

20. *Id.*, at 212; 79 S.Ct. 709.

21. *Smith v. Pro Football, Inc.*, 1978—2 Trade Cases (CCH) ¶ 62,338, at 76,031–76,032 (1978).

22. *Supra*, note 1.

23. *Cf., Feminist Women's Health Center, Inc. v. Mohammad*, 586 F.2d 530 (5th Cir. 1978).

24. *United States v. Colgate & Co.*, 250 U.S. 300, 39 S.Ct. 465 (1919).

25. *See, e.g., Fortner Enterprises, Inc. v. United States Steel Corp.*, 394 U.S. 495, 89 S.Ct. 1252 (1969).

26. 15 U.S.C. § 2.

27. *See, e.g., Berkey Photo, Inc. v. Eastman Kodak Co.*, Memorandum on Post-Trial Motions, Antitrust and Trade Reg. Rep. (BNA) No. 871, at E-2 (July 1978).

28. *United States v. Aluminum Co. of America*, 148 F.2d 416 (2d Cir. 1945).

29. *See, e.g., United States v. Grinnell Corp.*, 384 U.S. 563, 86 S.Ct. 1698 (1966), where an 87 percent market share was held to demonstrate monopoly power.

30. *See, e.g., American Tobacco Co. v. United States*, 328 U.S. 781, 66 S.Ct. 1125 (1946).

31. *United States v. Consolidated Packaging Corp.*, 575 F.2d 117, 126–127 (7th Cir. 1978).

32. 15 U.S.C. §§ 11, *et seq.*

33. 15 U.S.C. § 14.

34. *See, e.g., supra*, note 23.

35. *Cf., Standard Oil Co. of Calif. v. United States*, 337 U.S. 293 (1949), with *Tampa Elec. Co. v. Nashville Coal Co.*, 365 U.S. 320 (1961).

36. 15 U.S.C. § 18.

37. 15 U.S.C. § 19.

38. 15 U.S.C. § 13.

39. 15 U.S.C. §§ 41, *et seq.*

40. 15 U.S.C. § 45.

41. *Cf., Burch v. Goodyear Tire and Rubber Co.*, 420 F. Supp. 82 (D.C. Md. 1976).

42. *See, e.g., FTC v. Markin*, 391 F. Supp. 865 (D.C. Mich. 1974).

43. 15 U.S.C. § 46.

44. 15 U.S.C. § 44.

45. *Cf., Community Blood Bank of Kansas City Area v. FTC*, 405 F.2d 1011 (1969).

46. *Supra*, note 2.

47. *See, e.g., Goldfarb v. Virginia State Bar*, 421 U.S. 773, 95 S.Ct. 2004 (1975).

48. 425 U.S. 738, 96 S.Ct. 1848 (1976).

49. *Zamiri v. William Beaumont Hosp.*, 430 F. Supp. 875 (E.D. Mich. 1977).

50. American Medical Ass'n, *supra*, note 1.

51. *Cf., Willis v. Santa Ana Hosp. Ass'n,* 58 Cal.2d 806, 26 Cal.Rptr. 640 (1962), while this decision predates the Supreme Court's broadening of the Sherman Act, the general danger is that state courts will not immediately apply broader readings of the Sherman Act to state statutes.

52. *See, Datillo v. Tucson General Hosp.,* 23 Ariz.App. 392, 533 P.2d 700 (1975).

53. 15 U.S.C. § 17.

54. *See,* H.R. 13304 (95th Cong. 2d Sess.), introduced in the House of Representatives June 28, 1978.

55. 15 U.S.C. § 13(c).

56. 42 U.S.C. § 1320c–16(d)(1).

57. 421 U.S. 773, 95 S.Ct. 2004 (1975). See note 47, *supra.*

58. *National Soc'y of Professional Engineers v. United States,* 98 S.Ct. 1355 (1978).

59. *Illinois Brick Co. v. Illinois,* 431 U.S. 720, 97 S.Ct. 2061 (1977).

60. *See,* S. 300, the Antitrust Enforcement Act of 1979.

61. *Supra,* note 14, at 4; 78 S.Ct. 517 (1958).

Chapter 2

Antitrust Obstacles in Health Care

Until relatively recently the health care industry had been largely immune from both antitrust intervention and extensive government economic regulation. However, price competition in the industry has long been limited by the combined effects of state licensing laws, professional associations, and the inherent economic distinctiveness of "health care" as a commodity. In light of the traditional weakness of price competition in the health care market, with the precipitous rise in costs and the concomitant explosion of federally created entitlements, beginning with the Medicare and Medicaid Amendments of 1965,[1] it was inevitable that the industry's antitrust anonymity should come to an end.

As health care costs increased substantially faster than inflation, some antitrust enforcers concluded that, although the nature of the industry heretofore precluded effective price competition, aggressive application of the antitrust laws could be used to establish a competitive market that would have the eventual effect, under traditional economic theory, of controlling costs.[2] Thus, as the federal government strives to prevent the resulting drain on its available revenues from becoming prohibitively burdensome, it is not surprising that it should turn to the antitrust laws as ready-made weapons for the fight against spiraling health care costs.

However, the health care industry is characterized by significant economic peculiarities that make effective application of the antitrust laws more than ordinarily problematic. Ironically, other forms of government intervention are largely responsible for the industry's peculiarities. The nature of these peculiarities is the subject of this chapter.

The health care industry is different from the typical industry because of the interaction of two basic factors, one external and one internal. The external factor is increasingly extensive regulation by all levels of government; the internal factor is the economically anomalous nature of the health care market itself, which is, of course, interrelated with government regulation. Thus, a basic understanding of government regulation, the context within which the health care industry must operate, is an essential prerequisite to an understanding of the industry's peculiarities and of the consequent obstacles to the effective application of antitrust doctrine.

GOVERNMENT INTERVENTION IN THE HEALTH CARE INDUSTRY

The health care industry, according to government figures, is the third largest industry in the United States, employing well over 4.5 million persons.[3] Only agriculture and construction account for a larger percentage of the gross national product. Since 1950, health care spending has risen at four times the rate of inflation.[4] It is estimated that total national health care expenditures in 1980 will approach a quarter of a trillion dollars and, if the current rate of growth continues, will double in less than seven years.[5] Federal spending comprises nearly one-third of current health expenditures, paying over half of the country's yearly hospital care bill through Medicare, Medicaid, and other government programs.[6]

Increased government spending inevitably has meant increased government control. The health care industry has been called "the most highly regulated 'unregulated industry' in the country."[7] Regulation also affects other industries in areas such as civil rights, labor relations, occupational safety and health, taxes, and antitrust, but the health care industry faces an additional array of often bewilderingly complex programs that affect no other industry directly. Although government regulation in general has a significant impact on the health care industry, this chapter, because it is concerned with the peculiarities of the industry, will deal only with regulation aimed directly at the industry.

Federal Regulation: Medicare and Medicaid

The primary watershed in the history of federal spending on health occurred in 1965 with the passage of the Medicare and Medicaid Amendments to the Social Security Act.[8] Medicare, or Title XVIII of the Social Security Amendments of 1965, was created as a two-part program to provide health services to the aged and disabled. By 1972, almost all persons over the age of 65 were covered by Part A of Medicare,[9] which pays benefits for hospitalization and posthospitalization extended care and home health care through Social Security taxes paid by employers and employees. Part B, also known as Supplementary Medical Insurance, is an elective program covering physicians' fees as well as outpatient and diagnostic services, physical therapy, ambulance service, and other health care-related services not covered by Part A. Part B is financed in part by monthly premiums paid by the beneficiaries, with the federal government financing the remainder through general revenues.

Medicaid, or Title XIX of the Social Security Act of 1965, is a state-administered and partially state-financed program that provides health care benefits for the poor and the near-poor regardless of age. Reimbursement under Medicaid is on the basis of "reasonable cost," as defined by the states.

Medicare and Medicaid, conceived during a period of national economic growth and relative good health, became financially burdensome in an economic environment characterized by increasingly severe inflation. The government responded to the drain on its revenues from these two programs with regulations that, rather than limiting benefits, reduced reimbursement to providers. As a result, hospitals and other providers are paid on the basis of cost-reimbursement formulas that do not cover their actual expenditures. This method of reimbursement has had a profound effect on the health care market (discussed later in this chapter). For the purposes of this section, Medicare and Medicaid are particularly significant because they have cleared the way for increased government control of the health care industry. They are the carrot and the stick by which the government enforces restrictive regulatory programs.

Health Planning: P.L. 93-641

Health planning today represents government's attempt to control health care costs while maintaining both the availability of medical care to the needy and the quality of care in general. Health planners generally believe that unbridled competition, particularly among hospitals and particularly on the basis of quality rather than price, has brought about an oversupply of beds, physician specialists, and sophisticated equipment. The federal government has turned to health planning policy as a method of achieving its social goals without bankrupting itself, based on the premise that restricting the oversupply of medical services will reduce costs.

However, governmental health planning has not always been synonymous with restriction. Indeed, formal governmental health planning in the United States began as an attempt to remedy a perceived shortage and misallocation of hospital resources, with the Hill-Burton Hospital Survey and Construction Act of 1946.[10] Like Medicaid, the Hill-Burton program was established as a federal-state partnership in which state agencies were granted seed money to survey hospital needs and then carry out construction programs to meet those needs. By the end of 1974 (by which time amendments to the program had shifted its emphasis from grants to loans and loan guarantees), it was clear that the Hill-Burton program had succeeded in completely overcoming the post-World War II bed shortage; unfortunately, it had succeeded so well that there were approximately 40,000 surplus hospital beds in the United States.[11]

In response to the effects of Hill-Burton, Congress passed the second major federal health planning legislation, the Comprehensive Health Planning and Public Health Services Amendments of 1966,[12] which funded areawide Comprehensive Health Planning (CHP) agencies that were given responsibility for coordinating and controlling health care delivery. Although the areawide CHP agencies proved to be insufficiently funded and thus inadequately staffed, they also were required to review in detail significant capital expenditures by health facilities, under either Section 1122 of the Social Security Amendments of 1972 or state certificate of need laws.[13] In so doing, they were unable to develop the comprehensive health plans under which the expenditures were to be approved or rejected.[14] In response to these shortcomings, Congress passed the National Health Planning and Resources Development Act of 1974, also known as P.L. 93-641.[15]

P.L. 93-641 was a highly complex piece of legislation intended to remedy the deficiencies of the Comprehensive Health Planning Act of 1966 and, more generally, the "maldistribution of health care facilities and manpower and the lack of equal access to quality health care at a reasonable cost."[16] P.L. 93-641 thus represented a determination by the federal government that the health care market had failed either to contain costs or to distribute resources equitably and therefore must come under a significant measure of government control. The act was intended to eliminate from the health care market what were perceived as undesirable forms of competition, through multiinstitutional activities such as coordinated planning, group purchases, shared services, and other cost-limiting activities.

The act and the regulations developed under it have had a further restraining effect on competition by requiring that every state have a certificate of need law, whereby certain capital expenditures, including "[t]he construction, development or other establishment of a new health care facility or health maintenance organization,"[17] must be reviewed and may be prohibited (on pain of loss of Medicare and Medicaid reimbursement as well as other sanctions). The first level of such a certificate of need review is performed by a Health Systems Agency (HSA), a federally funded nonprofit corporation with semiregulatory powers over health care in a geographic area called a "health service area." In addition to performing certificate of need reviews, the HSA is required to review regularly all institutional health services in the area and to make recommendations to a designated state administrative agency concerning the "appropriateness" of these services.[18]

Finally, P.L. 93-641 requires that uniform cost accounting systems be developed, which has been seen as the first step toward effective rate regulation at the state level or under national health insurance.[19]

Health Services Delivery: The HMO Act of 1973

In addition to providing health services directly to patients felt to be served inadequately by private providers through federal hospitals or grants to the private sector, the federal government has attempted to promote the development of a new and possibly more efficient way of organizing and delivering health services: the Health Maintenance Organization (HMO).

The Federal Health Maintenance Organization Act of 1973[20] authorized $375 million to help finance HMOs. In addition, employers with more than 24 workers covered by the Fair Labor Standards Act were required to offer their employees the choice of an HMO, if one existed. By replacing the traditional fee-for-service basis on which most medical care is delivered with a fixed monthly fee, HMOs are intended to provide a previously absent incentive to control costs.[21] However, the health maintenance act also required HMOs to provide certain benefits that could be prohibitively expensive and to allow low-income and elderly patients to become members, despite the relatively high medical costs of such groups.

As a result, the development of the HMO, which HEW had announced in 1970 would be available to 90 percent of the population within ten years,[22] has been disappointing to its advocates.[23] Despite 1976 amendments to the act that were intended to overcome the handicaps,[24] highly restrictive qualification standards remain.[25] For this reason as well as others, the narrowed goal of the proponents of HMOs—to stimulate competition among health care providers—has not yet been realized.

Thus, it appears that the federal government's efforts to inject competition into the health care industry thus far have been even less effective than its attempts to restrain competition, although the HMOs' proponents still, perhaps not unreasonably, see it as the panacea for the competitive ills of the health care market.[26]

Regulation of Costs and Utilization: PSRO

Professional Standards Review Organizations (PSROs) were established on a national level under the Social Security Amendments of 1972[27] as a means of controlling the quality of health care as well as its costs. A PSRO generally is a nonprofit organization composed of physicians who work in the service area covered by the group. This organization either supervises or itself performs utilization review, which is intended to ensure the medical necessity, professional quality, and appropriate delivery of medical care.[28]

The utilization review concept grew out of the tissue committees established by the American College of Surgeons in 1949 to review the appropriateness of surgical operations.[29] In the early 1950s, the Joint Commission on Accreditation of Hospitals began to advocate the use of medical audits to assess the quality of care delivered in hospitals. By 1974, hospitals were required to have an appropriate medical audit procedure in effect as a condition of accreditation.[30] Utilization review committees were established under the requirements of the Medicare law as a condition of participation in that program.[31]

Under the 1972 legislation, a PSRO has the authority to perform utilization reviews of area hospitals or to delegate this function to each hospital's utilization review committee if the "delegated review" is deemed to be effective. But the authority of PSROs goes farther: they also are given responsibility to prepare standards and criteria to guide patient care. A PSRO decision that a particular treatment decision was inappropriate could result in loss of reimbursement for that service. Total exclusion from reimbursement under Medicare and Medicaid and up to $5,000 fines can be levied where violations are particularly egregious or numerous.[32]

To obtain the support of physicians, the PSRO program so far has emphasized improvement in the quality of care by physician self-regulation, rather than the PSROs' cost-limiting utilization control aspects.[33] Indeed, it has been suggested that the law's malpractice shield, which generally protects physicians who follow PSRO standards for malpractice liability, encourages increased utilization.[34] On balance, however, the backers of the program believe it will stimulate competition and thus reduce costs by disseminating general information on the performance of practitioners and providers to traditionally underinformed health care consumers.[35] Nevertheless, it is questionable whether a program that seeks to assure high quality medical care is likely to reduce costs.

The Future: Cost Containment and National Health Insurance

The most recent major development in federal regulation of health care has been the 1978 direct hospital cost containment legislation. Separate cost containment measures were introduced in the 95th Congress by Senator Herman E. Talmadge (D-Ga.) and the Carter Administration.[36] Although the bills were defeated by the strong lobbying of the American Medical Association, American Hospital Association, Federation of American Hospitals, and other representatives of the health care industry, and despite the immediate and not insubstantial preliminary success of the industry's "voluntary effort" program to hold down costs, which began in 1978, cost containment is likely to remain a major legislative issue as long as health care costs continue to rise faster than the rate of inflation. It appears that some additional federal cost containment legislation will be adopted in the near future and probably will result in further profound effects on the industry.

Because of public concern over inflation, particularly in regard to health care costs, passage of a national health insurance program (NHI) was somewhat less likely, although some form of partial national health insurance, such as comprehensive catastrophic coverage, might be adopted. However, cost containment legislation, the National Health Planning and Resources Development Act of

1974, the tightening of Medicare and Medicaid reimbursement rules, and the PSRO and HMO laws all were regarded as preparatory programs by the federal government to clear the way for a full-fledged NHI program.[37] It remained to be seen whether that goal ever would be realized, but if it were to be, all of these programs might not be able to control the resulting costs.

The reasons for this are two. First, a 1974 study by the Rand Corporation predicted that NHI, while limiting the demand for hospital-based care, would cause a precipitous increase in the demand for ambulatory care.[38] The preparatory programs cited shared this bias against hospitals because they were based on the federal government's experience with Medicare, which brought about greatly increased hospital use and therefore higher hospital costs.[39] Second, history indicates any NHI program, such as Social Security, Medicare, and Medicaid, and numerous other past federal subsidy efforts, probably will incur substantial, ever-increasing costs, resulting in new demands for further government action. At that point, the choice may be between significant deregulation (along with, it is likely, stepped-up antitrust enforcement) on the one hand and socialized medicine on the other.

State and Local Regulation

Regulation at the state and local government level in many respects is similar to federal regulation. First, there is considerable regulation not aimed specifically at the health care industry but affecting it along with other industries, from local zoning ordinances to state statutes and regulations on civil rights, antitrust, and other areas also covered by federal law. Several of the programs discussed above are funded at least in part by the federal government but administered largely at the state level. These include Medicaid, certificate of need review and planning by Health Systems Agencies under the National Health Planning and Resources Development Act of 1974, and Section 1122 capital expenditure review under the Social Security Amendments of 1972. There are, however, two major activities that states perform largely autonomously, the first traditional—licensing—and the second a relatively recent regulatory development—rate review.

State Licensing

Although every state requires a license to practice medicine, it is not totally accurate to call the licensing requirements state regulation. In practice, state licensing means professional self-regulation by the health care industry of its members, from major hospitals to veterinarians. Administrative agencies traditionally become close to the industries they regulate,[40] but no industry has exerted more control over the regulatory process than the health care industry. In part, this control has resulted from the highly technical nature of the field. Perhaps a more important reason for regulators' acquiescence to the industry's dominance of the licensing process is the high esteem in which members of the medical profession traditionally have been held by the public. Unlike the usual regulated businesses, health care providers have been viewed as concerned with the saving of lives and the alleviation of suffering rather than profits and power. This view has begun to break down, however, under the pressure of mounting costs and the consequent increase in criticism of health care providers.

The licensing aspect of the health care industry is particularly vulnerable to antitrust intervention because it often has the anticompetitive effect of creating both direct and indirect barriers to entry into the field. An example of an indirect barrier that results from state licensing is medical school accreditation by the American Medical Association (AMA). Since most states require graduation from an AMA-accredited medical school, the organization indirectly controls entry into the medical profession.[41] In practice, the effect of AMA accreditation has been to limit the number of medical schools (which remain fewer in number today than when the AMA first began to control accreditation in the early 1900s)[42] and to raise medical school entrance and graduation requirements that, like licensing itself, have been justified as necessary to ensure high quality medical care and to protect patients from incompetent practitioners.[43]

By the late 1960s, however, another effect was perceived: a shortage of physicians.[44] This problem came to be viewed as one of physician maldistribution rather than a real shortage.[45] In fact, it was estimated that by 1980 there would be one physician for every 490 persons in the country—the highest level of physicians since the beginning of the twentieth century.[46] There is little doubt that barriers to entry, however justifiable, have helped to keep physicians' fees high. Moreover, licensing has limited severely or precluded entry into the health care field by medical personnel who may be capable of performing procedures for which an M.D. is not essential, which could reduce the costs of medical care.[47] State nursing practice acts, for example, not only have restricted the procedures that may be performed by otherwise capable nurses, but also have required that many procedures that nurses may perform be controlled and supervised by physicians. All of these aspects of licensing are being examined closely by both the Federal Trade Commission and the Justice Department's Antitrust Division.[48]

Rate Review

As of the end of 1978, 27 states had some form of hospital budget or rate review program, which may be defined as "any committee or board which prospectively monitors, reviews or establishes the rates, charges, cost or revenue of a group of health care institutions."[49] A budget/rate review program generally is administered either by a state agency or Blue Cross.[50] While six of these programs were merely advisory in nature, in that the administrative body had no authority to determine or change rates and had no power to sanction recalcitrant providers,[51] the remaining 21 programs, covering approximately 2,100 hospitals, were full-fledged budget or rate regulation operations.[52]

Budget/rate review programs are a relatively new development in state regulation of the industry; only two states had such a program before 1971.[53] Regulation of hospital rates has become an increasingly popular state-level response to perceived health care costs. As of mid-1979, of the 22 states that lacked some form of budget/rate review program, at least 15 were considering starting one.[54] With health care costs unlikely to abate in the near future, such budget/rate review programs probably will continue to proliferate.

THE ABERRATIONAL ECONOMICS OF THE HEALTH CARE INDUSTRY

Most of the regulation discussed in the previous section is premised on the assumption that the health care market does not function the way a market is supposed to, that the "Alice in Wonderland economics of health care"[55] has virtually eliminated effective price competition. Indeed, the health care market deviates substantially in many major respects from the norms of classic economic market theory. In a perfectly competitive market, consumers choose which goods to purchase on the basis of informed judgments. In the health care market, it generally is believed that consumers lack adequate information about products and services. A commentator has stated:

> The nature of health care is such that the consumer knows very little about the medical services he or she is buying. . . . Some choices about medical care are made solely by patients. But a very large part of the decision making is done by physicians—diagnosis, treatment, drugs and tests, hospitalization, frequency of return visits are all substantially under the physician's control. . . . While the consumer can participate in policing the market, that participation is much more limited than in almost any other area of private economic activity.[56]

This information deficiency has not resulted from a conspiracy on the part of health care providers to keep consumers ignorant regarding the nature and comparative quality of available forms of medical care. This problem in part is a result of the very complexity of the practice of medicine. Even with a thorough understanding of medicine, however,[57] consumers still would have difficulty obtaining sufficient information upon which to base reasoned purchase decisions because they could not judge accurately what has been called the "counterfactual"—the result of not purchasing care.[57]

[A] consumer of such services who gets better after the purchase does not know whether the improvement was because of, or even in spite of, the "care" that was received. Or if no health care services are purchased and the individual's problem becomes worse, he is generally not in a strong position to determine whether the results would have been better . . . if he had purchased certain health care . . . The noteworthy point is not simply that it is difficult for the consumer to judge quality before the purchase (as it also is in the [purchase of a] used car . . .), but that it is difficult even after the purchase.[58]

As a result of their relative ignorance, patients exert minimal influence over the amount, kind, and quality of medical care services they purchase; these decisions instead are made by physicians. Thus, demand in the health care market, as opposed to other markets where the consumer is said to be "sovereign," is determined to a substantial extent by the market's sellers rather than its buyers.[59]

Physicians have significant control not only over the demand for medical care but also over the supply. As discussed earlier in regard to state licensing, self-regulation by the health care industry has resulted in direct and indirect barriers to entry into the market and generally has limited competition, particularly among physicians, by such means as advertising restrictions, denial of medical staff privileges, exclusive hospital contracts, specialist certification, and relative value scales.

Many commentators have concluded that the basic form of active competition in the health care industry is based on quality rather than price. Although in part this is due to the "priceless" nature of "good health," the major reason for the relative absence of price competition is the third-party payment system. Government programs, led by Medicare and Medicaid, and private insurers pay more than 90 percent of the total bill for hospital services. As a result, consumers generally need not consider price in deciding which medical services to purchase, and therefore it largely is unnecessary for providers to compete on the basis of price. Despite the much discussed health care cost crisis, consumers' actual out-of-pocket health care expenses have risen at a rate lower than the general national rate of inflation.[60]

Presumably, therefore, the third-party payment system has stimulated consumer demand, thereby driving up prices. In addition, hospitals are reimbursed by third-party payors on the basis of costs incurred in patient care, which also leads to higher prices by providing an incentive for inefficiency and, because such reimbursement often does not cover actual hospital costs fully, by forcing hospitals to increase rates to patients who pay directly for services in order to offset losses from third-party payments.[61]

Although it theoretically is possible for these third-party payors themselves to exert bargaining and purchasing power to help contain costs, the incentive to exert such power depends upon the independence and financial motivation of the purchasers, and the major third-party payors—Blue Cross and Blue Shield— have been accused of being dominated by and thus beholden to the health care industry.[62]

Another important difference between the health care market and other markets is the prevalence of nonprofit entities, which sometimes are assumed, whether properly or not, to be less competitive. This assumption is based on the following analysis:

> The profit motive encourages technical efficiency and low-cost production. The marketplace disciplines firms that become overly inefficient. Nonprofit producers, however, do not have the same pressures for efficient production nor the same incentives to adjust output in order to achieve higher profit.[63]

In reply, however, it has been argued that nonprofit institutions are beneficial socially, particularly as they use their positions to generate the funds needed to provide care for the indigent.[64]

Finally, as noted, many observers have concluded that health care providers compete largely on the basis of quality, which is described as "the antithesis of price competition . . . founded on the virtual disregard for price made possible by third-party payment methods."[65] Quality at the hospital level sometimes is equated with advanced technology, which is the primary basis for competition among hospitals, which thereby compete indirectly for patients by competing for physicians to be members of their medical staffs.[66] In so doing, however, their defenders argue that hospitals merely are responding to consumer demand, which is particularly strong because, as noted, it is relatively unfettered by cost restraints as a result of the third-party payment system and because of the uniquely overriding importance of health to the consumer. As one commentator has stated:

> All the people who are worried about a multibillion-dollar health bill also want their hip replaced when they fall down, their coronary bypass surgery when they have angina pain, their kidneys transplanted and their leukemia treated by the most effective means. We can make some cuts, but I don't think we can stop medical costs from going up.[67]

This brief summary of the health care industry's unique aspects is intended to provide a basis for understanding the reasons that those responsible for enforcing the antitrust laws have turned their attention toward this industry as well as the substantial difficulties and thorny policy issues included in the application of those laws to the industry. Antitrust doctrine is not inflexible, and the peculiarities of the health care industry should affect the way the traditional rules are applied, particularly where assumptions that may be made about other industries are inapplicable.

NOTES

1. Pub. L. 89-97, Titles XVIII and XIX of the Social Security Amendments of 1965.

2. *See Health Lawyers News Report* (February 1979); *PSRO Letter* (Jan. 15, 1979), at 2–3; *Group Practice* (May-June 1978), at 8–11.

3. *U.S. News & World Report* (March 5, 1979), at 33.

4. *Id.,* at 40.

5. *Id.,* at 33.

6. *Id.,* at 33, 40; U.S. Department of Health, Education, and Welfare, Social Security Administration, *Medical Care Expenditures, Prices and Costs: Background Book,* (1975).

7. Coopers & Lybrand, *A Layman's Guide to Hospitals* (1978), at 19. *See generally,* A. Somers and H. Somers, *Health and Health Care: Policies in Perspective,* 239–275 (Aspen Systems, 1977).

8. 42 U.S.C. §§ 1395, 1396 (Supp. V 1975).

9. U.S. Department of Health, Education, and Welfare, Social Security Administration, *Medicare: Health Insurance for the Aged,* 1972, HEW Publication No. (SSA) 75-11704 (1975).

10. Pub. L. 79-725 (1946).

11. U.S. Department of Health, Education, and Welfare, Public Health Services, Health Resources Administration, *Trends Affecting U.S. Health Care System* 94 (1975) (hereinafter Trends).

12. Pub. L. 89-749, 42 U.S.C. §§ 1320a-1, 1320c to 1320c-19 (Supp. V 1975).

13. Trends, at 98.

14. *Id.,* at 99.

15. 42 U.S.C. §§ 300k *et seq.* (Supp. V 1975).

16. 42 U.S.C. § 300k-2(1) and (a)(3)(B), respectively.

17. 42 Fed. Reg. 4002, 4025, 4029 (1977).

18. *See generally,* "Symposium: Certificate of Need Laws in Health Planning," 1978 *Utah L. Rev.* 1.

19. Trends, at 108.

20. Pub. L. 93-222, 42 U.S.C. §§ 280c, 300c to 300e-14a (Supp. III 1973).

21. H. Somers, "Health and Public Policy" *Inquiry,* Vol. XII, No. 2, 87–96, reprinted in *Economics in Health Care* 13–22 (Aspen Systems 1975).

22. *Id.,* at 15.

23. Trends, at 242.

24. Pub. L. 94-460; 42 U.S.C. §§ 300e *et seq.*

25. C. Havighurst, "Health Maintenance Organizations and the Health Planners," 1978 *Utah L. Rev.* at 123, 135.

26. *See, e.g.,* D. Drake and D. Kozak, "A Price on Antitrust Hospital Regulation," *J. of Health Pol. Pol'y L.,* (Fall 1978), at 337–338; *see generally, The Health Maintenance Organization and Its Effects on Competition* (Federal Trade Commission 1975).

27. Pub. L. 92-602, 42 U.S.C. §§ 1320e *et seq.*

28. *Competition in the Health Care Sector: Past, Present and Future* (Federal Trade Commission 1978), at 106 (hereinafter FTC).

29. Trends, at 131–132.

30. *Id.*, at 132.

31. *Id.*

32. *Id.*, at 134.

33. FTC, at 108.

34. *Id.*, at 109.

35. *Id.*, at 109–110.

36. The 1978 bills were S. 1470 and S. 1391, respectively.

37. Trends, at 130.

38. J. Newhouse, C. Phelps, W. Schwartz, *Policy Options and the Impact of National Insurance* (1974).

39. Trends, at 131.

40. *See* M. Bernstein, *Regulating Business by Independent Commission* (1955).

41. M. Cane, "Restrictive Practices in Accreditation of Medical Schools: An Antitrust Analysis," 51 *So. Cal. L. Rev.* 657, 658 (1978); R. Kessel, "The AMA and the Supply of Physicians," 35 *Law & Contemp. Prob.* 267, 268 (1970); Rayack, "Restrictive Practices in Organized Medicine," 13 *Antitrust Bull.* 659, 664 (1968); Comment, "The American Medical Association: Power, Purpose and Politics in Organized Medicine, 63 *Yale L.J.* 938, 969 (1954).

42. Cane, *supra* note 4, at 658, n 8.

43. R. Stevens, *American Medicine and the Public Interest* 68 (1971).

44. Kessel, *supra*, note 4 at 268.

45. J. Lister, "How Many Doctors," *New England J. of Med.*, 1215–1217 (May 26, 1977); C. Stewart, Jr., and C. Siddayau, *Increasing the Supply of Medical Personnel: Needs and Alternatives* (American Enterprise Institute 1973).

46. *U.S. News & World Report, supra*, note 3, at 40.

47. "Antitrust and Medicine: A Justice Department Perspective," *Group Practice* (May-June 1978), at 10.

48. *Id.*

49. American Hospital Ass'n, "Report on Budget/Rate Review Programs" (1978), at 1.

50. *Id.*, at 10.

51. *Id.*, at 8.

52. *Id.*

53. *Id.*, at 3–7.

54. *Id.*, at 14.

55. *U.S. News & World Report, supra*, note 3, at 35.

56. K. Davis, "Economic Theories of Behavior in Nonprofit Private Hospitals," *J. of Econ. and Bus.* (Winter 1972), quoted in M. Pauly, "Is Medical Care Different," in FTC, at 23.

57. B. Weisbrod, "Comment," in FTC, at 52.

58. *Id.*

59. *See generally*, F. Sloan and R. Feldman, "Competition Among Physicians," in FTC, at 57–131.

60. Drake and Kozak, *supra*, note 26, at 334.

61. Coopers & Lybrand, *supra*, note 7, at 18.

62. *See, e.g.*, C. Weller, "Medicaid Boycotts and Other Maladies from Medical Monopolists: An Introduction to Antitrust Litigation and the Health Care Industry," 11 *Clearinghouse Review* 99,100 (June 1977).

63. J. Blumstein and F. Sloan, "Efficiency, Incentives and Reimbursement for Health Care," 7 *Inquiry* 114 (1978), at 4, citing Pauly.

64. C. Havighurst, "Health Maintenance Organizations and the Market for Health Services," 35 *Law & Contemp. Prob.* 716 (1970) (hereinafter Havighurst).

65. *Id.*, at 336.

66. J. Blumstein and F. Sloan, "Health Planning and Regulation Through Certificate of Need: An Overview," 1978 *Utah L. Rev.* 3, 5 (hereinafter Blumstein and Sloan).

67. Dr. Robert Heyssel, director of Johns Hopkins Hospital, Baltimore, quoted in *U.S. News & World Report*, *supra*, note 3, at 36.

Chapter 3

Health Planning and Other Government Interventions

The impact of both involuntary government intervention in health care and voluntary use of governmental resources by providers raises issues regarding the interaction between and among statutes and policies other than, and sometimes inconsistent with, the antitrust laws. This chapter explores the antitrust exemptions and immunities, as well as potential liability, created through the interaction of government regulations, regulators, and tribunals with health care providers. The analysis is subdivided to consider the markedly different exemptions and immunities applicable, first, to those occasions on which providers, including organized groups, voluntarily seek to influence governmental decision-making processes and, second, to the occasions when government regulation of the industry results in conduct inconsistent with ordinary antitrust principles.

PROVIDER EFFORTS TO INFLUENCE OFFICIALS' CONDUCT

The health care industry must deal with, and depend upon, the almost daily decisions of officials at all levels of government:

1. the federal government in determining and enacting federal policies on health planning and on reimbursement
2. state governments in establishing and implementing mechanisms for complying (or determining not to comply) with federal policies, as well as in determining the states' own independent health planning and reimbursement policies and mechanisms
3. local governments in obtaining city and county zoning, planning, and environmental approval
4. local health systems agencies and state health planning agencies in reaching individual planning (certificate of need and certificate of exemption) decisions

5. each level of government as a potential or actual purchaser of health care
   services

The conduct of government officials in establishing and implementing policies, in reaching individual decisions to grant or deny necessary certificates or to
reimburse for services supplied through subsidized programs, and in purchasing
services from providers, have major financial impact and may even mean the
difference between functioning as a provider and ceasing (or never commencing)
to function. Consequently, the need to deal effectively within these governmental processes and the incentives and opportunities for abuses of the systems,
often for directly anticompetitive purposes, are correspondingly significant.

It is fortunate that the courts have recognized broad protections from antitrust
prosecution for efforts to influence governmental action toward anticompetitive
results. It also is fortunate that they have provided detailed explanations and
guidance regarding the parameters of the protected conduct. To describe and
analyze properly what conduct is protected, and to distinguish that conduct from
what goes beyond the limits of immunity, it is necessary first to classify provider
influence over governmental conduct into three functional categories, each of
which receives varying degrees of immunities:

1. efforts to influence governmental policy-making decisions
2. efforts to influence government adjudications in individually applying established policies, laws, and regulations
3. efforts to influence government purchasing decisions

Influencing Government Policy-Making Decisions

Perhaps the most complete subordination of the policies of the antitrust laws
in promoting competition and prohibiting concerted action to eliminate competitors or create monopolies is found in the resolution of the conflict between those
policies and the First Amendment rights of freedom of speech, association, and
to petition the government on policy determinations. In general, where citizens—
even groups of competitors acting jointly—actually are seeking to influence governmental policy decisions of a legislative nature, their First Amendment rights,
together with the need for government to receive information (whether accurate,
honest, or otherwise), have been considered too important and too sensitive to
be chilled by even the threat of antitrust prosecution based upon the anticompetitive motives behind the exercise of those rights.

The basic rule explaining the subordination of antitrust principles to First
Amendment rights was established by the Supreme Court in a 1961 case titled
Eastern Railway Presidents Conference v. Noerr Motor Freight, Inc.,[1] which
involved government regulation of long-distance freight hauling by both the

trucking and railroad industries. In this situation, a group of trucking companies, together with their trade association, had sued 24 railroads and a public relations firm, charging that they had conspired to restrain trade to monopolize the long-distance freight business in violation of Sections 1 and 2 of the Sherman Act. The plaintiffs contended that the restraint of trade was effected through the mechanism of a concerted publicity campaign against the truckers, by and on behalf of the railroads. The railroads were accused of a "vicious, corrupt, and fraudulent" campaign for the sole purpose of injuring the truckers and destroying them as competitors. The truckers charged that the railroads had succeeded in influencing the governor of Pennsylvania to veto a bill that would have extended the rights of truckers to compete more effectively with the railroads by carrying heavier loads over the Commonwealth's roads.

The railroads essentially admitted they had undertaken the publicity campaign to influence the passage of state laws on truck weight limits and tax rates. They contended, however, that they were within their rights in informing the public and the legislatures of the damages being caused by trucks' hauling of heavy freight.

The Supreme Court issued an opinion which now affects, and may even shape, activities in every industry—not the least of which is the health care industry—that regularly depends upon government. Starting with a basic construction of the Sherman Act that excluded attempts to influence the passage or enforcement of laws from the purview of the act, the court explained that where a restraint of trade or monopolization resulted from valid governmental action, the act remained inapplicable. Reaching the more involved questions presented by the conduct in *Noerr,* the court said the mere fact that a group of competitors had joined together to influence governmental action could not make the Sherman Act applicable where it otherwise was not. In fact, the court held, the functioning of a democratic government often depends upon associations of persons making their wishes known to their representatives. It also found no indication that Congress had intended to invade the right of individuals to petition their government.

The court said the breadth of the exemption from antitrust liability in this type of activity made the motive for seeking to influence governmental action essentially inconsequential. It is only realistic to assume that persons who seek to influence the government will do so for their own benefit, and it occasionally follows that obtaining such a benefit requires conduct to the disadvantage of a competitor, the court declared. It said that to eliminate the solicitation of governments whenever that action was for such an anticompetitive purpose would deprive the officials of a valuable source of information and create an unwarranted infringement on the right of persons to petition their governments. Although the truckers also alleged that the railroads' publicity campaign involved unethical business conduct and the deception of the public through the use of misleading reference sources and the distortion of information, the court chose to leave the resolution of such problems to ordinary political processes or, at most, to judicial processes without the assistance of the antitrust laws.

In considering the truckers' contention that the railroads' publicity campaign had interfered directly with the trucking business, not through influencing government action but through deception of the public, the court explained the one basic exception to the exemption from antitrust prosecution it was then creating. Known as the "sham" exception, this provides that where the challenged activity is not actually being used with a view toward influencing governmental action, but in effect is a mere sham to conceal an attempt to interfere directly with the business of a competitor, then the purpose for the First Amendment exception from the antitrust laws was lost, as was the exemption.[2] The court held, however, that publicity campaigns actually directed toward influencing governmental action could have the incidental effect of interfering with a competitor's business, as the public necessarily was informed of the position of those seeking to influence the government. This incidental effect, where the publicity campaign is not a mere sham but in reality is directed toward influencing governmental conduct, does not justify the application of the antitrust laws, the court ruled.

The breadth of the antitrust exemption established in the *Noerr* case was extended by the court in 1965 in *United Mine Workers of America v. Pennington*,[3] which involved an alleged conspiracy between certain coal mine operators and a miners union to cause the wages paid to miners to be set at a level so artificially high as to purposely put small mining companies out of business. Although the overall conspiracy was alleged to have been effectuated through various mechanisms, most of which enjoyed no immunities from antitrust prosecution, the court held that one aspect of the conspiracy was immune from antitrust attack. This consisted of the combination of the larger coal mine operators together with the union attempting to induce the U.S. Secretary of Labor to establish a minimum wage for employees of operators that sold coal to the Tennessee Valley Authority, the wage being at a level difficult for small companies to pay and thus helping to drive them out of business. The court succinctly applied the antitrust immunity established in *Noerr*, stating:

> Joint efforts to influence public officials do not violate the antitrust laws even though intended to eliminate competition. Such conduct is not illegal, either standing alone or as part of a broader scheme itself violative of the Sherman Act.[4]

The court, however, suggested a possible caveat from the immunity:

> The conduct of the union and the operators did not violate the [Sherman] Act, the action taken to set a minimum wage for government purchases

of coal was the act of a public official who is not claimed to be a co-conspirator. . .[5]

To this point, then, a broad exemption from antitrust principles had been created, allowing joint and concerted efforts among those who chose to combine and conspire to force competitors out of business through influence over governmental conduct, with the potential caveats that the apparent efforts to influence that conduct must not be a sham, calculated only to interfere directly with the business of the competitor, and the government officials at whom the influential activities were directed not be coconspirators. This basic exemption, known as the Noerr-Pennington doctrine, has been applied in numerous industries, generally with a very broad scope in order to exempt from antitrust scrutiny even what might appear to be blatantly abusive, unethical, and dishonest conduct.

In various contexts, attempts to lobby and petition local government agencies (acting in legislative capacities) to cause the denials of permits needed by potential competitors, with the result of denying such persons the opportunity to compete, have been held to be immune from antitrust attack. This immunity has not been lost or affected by the fact that those who conducted a lobbying campaign may have engaged in major distortions and misrepresentations of fact before the government agency. In fact, where the efforts to influence the agency involve a direct lobbying effort, it is virtually inconceivable that the immunity could be lost. Such a lobbying campaign should not reach the public, could not interfere directly with the business of the disadvantaged party, and consequently would not appear to be reasonably subject to allegations of being a sham.[6]

Even where those who seek to restrain trade succeed in causing the adoption of a law that itself is unconstitutional, the immunity from antitrust prosecution is not forfeited.[7] The First Amendment protection necessary to allow citizens freely to petition their government, for whatever reason, is too important and too sensitive to be chilled by a rule requiring those citizens to predict accurately the constitutionality of the legislation they promote. Nor is the immunity lost where the efforts to influence the government are carried out through economic coercion over the officials involved, as opposed to influence through arguments relating more directly to the merits of the requested conduct.[8]

The occasions on which the application of these general rules (relating to the legislative arena only) may become of interest to health care providers may be more extensive than the term "legislative" at first would indicate. To come within the immunity for efforts to influence legislative conduct, one need not be attempting to influence any legislator. Even local governmental units (such as a local Health Systems Agency) and state administrative agencies (including state health planning agencies) may be delegated the legislative power to reach policy decisions. For example, health planning agencies may act in a legislative capacity in setting policies that will determine boundaries of various health service areas, in establishing criteria for use in reaching decisions on certificate of need applications, and in setting procedures for committees to follow in hearing such applications.

Providers who succeed in influencing the outcome of any of these policy decisions may succeed thereby in assuring the outcome of subsequent certificate of need applications, perhaps making the actual hearing process for later applications a virtual nullity. The motivation for such influential activities could well include, and perhaps even be limited to, the goal of restricting the expansion of competitors, eliminating potential entry into the market, and maintaining a monopoly in a market.

A directly analogous situation was addressed by a federal appellate court with respect to a cable television market in Illinois.[9] Illinois state law had delegated to cities the legislative power to reach decisions on cable television services within their limits. A cable television company, together with an affiliate company and several individuals, successfully undertook a concerted effort to cause the Rockford city council to decide to grant only a single cable TV franchise in that city and to decide not to hold hearings on issuance of the franchise. Consequently, that particular company enjoyed a government-created monopoly in that area, and potential competitors were denied a formal hearing process to challenge that monopoly.

If the allegations of the plaintiff in this case, a rival cable television company directly disadvantaged by the city council's decision, are taken as true, the successful conspiracy had been effectuated through blatantly unethical and dishonest tactics. Not only had the successful company and coconspirators influenced the city council through erroneous statements of purported facts, they had enlisted the services of the mayor, through large campaign contributions, to use his own suasion over the city council and to make false filings with the Federal Communications Commission, the plaintiff charged.

The court, however, applied the broadest of the First Amendment exemptions from antitrust attacks and held that all of the conduct allegedly undertaken by the conspirators was immune. The court ruled that the city council's decision not to hold hearings did not exclude the unsuccessful contenders from the political processes, but merely forced them to approach the council through lobbying and means ordinarily associated with attempts to influence legislative (as opposed to adjudicatory) governmental units. The city council was not set up to operate as an adjudicative body, was not required to compile a formal record before acting, and could act on any informal information it might receive, the court said, adding that the denial of hearings could not bring the challenged conduct within the sham exception to the Noerr-Pennington immunity.

The impact of the mayor's involvement in the influencing of the defendant company presented a more sensitive question and one likely to be of repeated concern for health care providers who on occasion may enjoy close relations with local politicians. Although the court adopted language sometimes demeaning the notion that the involvement of government officials in a conspiracy may abrogate the otherwise available immunity, it was careful to explain that the mayor (and a city alderman accused of similar conduct) was not the governmental agency that reached the anticompetitive decision. Rather, the court decided, the mayor was only using his incidental capacity to assist in reaching the monopolistic result, through suasion of the city council. Moreover, to conclude that giving campaign contributions with a view toward gaining anticompetitive favors causes a loss of the right to petition and influence politicians freely would be to disregard an accepted (if not favored) part of the political process, the court said.

The question of the impact of involving governmental officials in the conspiracy itself, as opposed to their roles solely as objects of influential activities, has been the subject of some dispute, and has not been addressed authoritatively by the Supreme Court. As mentioned, the court left the question open to some extent in the *Pennington* (coal) case. In the celebrated *Rex Hospital* case,[10] the court explained in detail how conspiratorial efforts to use the health planning processes to obstruct the construction of a new hospital could affect the flow of interstate commerce sufficiently to subject the conspirators to the federal jurisdiction of the Sherman Act. The substantive allegations in that case involved a conspiracy that included a local health planning official as a coconspirator. Although the Supreme Court's jurisdictional decision did not reach the merits of the substantive allegations, if the court were to be called upon later to rule on the merits of this or a similar situation, the opinion could well be significantly enlightening.

Lacking the unifying influence of a detailed explanation from the Supreme Court, some lower courts have endeavored to develop the Noerr-Pennington immunity doctrine further in its application to conspiracies that include government agents among their coconspirators, with less than consistent results. The Court of Appeals for the Third Circuit, for example, ruled explicitly that the Noerr-Pennington immunity for efforts to influence government officials was not applicable where government officials actually participated with private persons in a scheme to restrain trade. The court held, in essence, that the Noerr-Pennington immunity was limited to occasions when the public body was acting within its legal discretion and in what it considered to be the public interest. However, where the public body itself collaborates to actually promote the anticompetitive conspiracy, the appellate court ruled, the otherwise available immunity is lost.[11]

The Court of Appeals for the Ninth Circuit, however, changed its own position from one similar to the Third Circuit's to one granting broader immunity, even where governmental officials participated in the conspiracy.[12]

It would appear now that the involvement of government agents, as actual "participants and coconspirators" rather than merely as the objects of the influential activities, is a dangerous course at best. Where government officials participate in an anticompetitive conspiracy, presumably for their direct or indirect personal gain, much of the rationale justifying the Noerr-Pennington immunity is rendered meaningless. The incidence of public office should not, and at this time apparently need not, immunize the anticompetitive conduct of the office-holder or the coconspirators who act with the official to disadvantage a rival. A contrary conclusion would allow the immunity to sanction a new type of sham conduct, whereby public officials could combine and conspire with others to serve their own ends and then seek the shelter of the merely incidental capacity of "public official" on the part of one coconspirator. Again, this situation must be distinguished from a properly immunized conspiracy that solicits the favor of the public official in seeking government action toward anticompetitive ends.

Efforts To Influence Adjudicatory Decisions

The courts have restricted the scope of the basic First Amendment, Noerr-Pennington immunity doctrine substantially when the anticompetitive efforts are directed toward influencing the decision of adjudicatory governmental bodies as opposed to legislative or policy-making bodies. Consequently, health care providers who seek to use state or federal courts, or administrative tribunals such as certificate of need hearing bodies, for anticompetitive purposes (such as joint opposition to a certificate of need application by a group of rival providers) should do so with circumspection in view of the increased possibilities of committing actionable antitrust violations. This is true particularly where the anticompetitive effort may involve the creation of delays or procedural roadblocks in the applicant's use of the adjudicative processes and where the opponents may envision the use of misstatements of fact and other unethical conduct. While such reprehensible tactics may be immunized in the legislative arena, they may form the basis for actionable, nonexempt violations of the antitrust laws when perpetrated in courtroom or administrative trial settings.

Here, again, the extensive regulation of the trucking industry (which in some respects is similar to that of the health care industry, as truckers depend upon the decisions of administrative tribunals for permission to operate new routes) caused the Supreme Court in 1972 for the first time to address the extent of immunities available for concerted, anticompetitive conduct before adjudicatory tribunals in the context of a dispute between truckers over their operating rights.[13] In the *Trucking, Unlimited* case, one group of truckers charged that another group had combined and conspired to restrain trade and monopolize certain transportation markets. The plaintiffs alleged that the conspiracy was effectuated through proceedings before administrative and judicial tribunals (regulatory hearing agencies and courts) to resist and defeat their applications for operating rights. The activities extended beyond the original hearing proceedings into the use of rehearings and appeals from court decisions, all of which caused great delays during which the truckers who required new operating rights could not function, the suit contended.

The Supreme Court ruled that the right of persons to join together to influence governmental adjudicatory bodies, even for the purpose of causing the agencies to reach decisions that would be destructive of the operating rights of actual or potential competitors, enjoyed a First Amendment protection (essentially to protect the right of association and to petition the government) and immunity from antitrust prosecution, similar in purpose to the immunity available for petitioning and influencing legislative bodies. The extent of the immunity here, however, is somewhat more circumscribed than that available in the legislative context.

The Supreme Court declared that where the conspiracy to restrain trade through the use of adjudicatory tribunals did not consist of efforts actually to influence the decisions of the tribunals, but rather of efforts to usurp the decision-making process by barring the competitors from meaningful access to the tribunals, then the immunity was lost. For example, the court explained, where the conspirators instituted a series of baseless actions, without regard for their merits, it may appear that the actions were not begun to take advantage of governmental decision-making processes, but only to discourage the competitors from themselves invoking the decision-making processes.

Of even greater significance, and almost certainly leading to greater eventual controversy, the Supreme Court commented specifically that misrepresentations and unethical conduct that might be tolerated in the legislative context could not be immunized when used in an adjudicatory process. Such unethical conduct often leads to other forms of sanctions when perpetrated before the courts, and the court concluded that the addition of the antitrust sanction is not significantly chilling to the exercise of any First Amendment right.

Consequently, the court established the rule that persons could join together to use administrative hearing bodies and the courts to defeat applications of competitors for operating certificates, and that a mere anticompetitive or even monopolistic purpose or effect would not abrogate the immunity. However, the court added, where the combination of competitors acts to harass and deter others from free and unlimited access to the agencies and courts, including a pattern of baseless actions or abuse of the judicial processes, then the immunity may be lost.[14]

The importance of this rule to providers who depend upon the health planning process should be apparent immediately. The advent of the certificate of need (and occasionally the certificate of exemption from certificate of need requirements) has made providers singularly dependent upon favorable administrative adjudicatory decisions, and sometimes upon favorable judicial determinations on appeal from administrative hearings. Where rival providers may seek to preserve their market position through concerted opposition to a certificate of need application, they will depend upon their First Amendment rights and consequent antitrust immunities. Their conduct in presenting and pursuing their concerted opposition, however, must be scrutinized carefully.

Because health planning agencies frequently (perhaps universally) depend upon the utilization, patient origin, capacity, and other statistics relating to, and often available only from, rivals of the certificate of need applicant, these rivals are given additional opportunities to disadvantage the applicant should their statistics indicate the planning impropriety of the project under review. A close analogy to this type of situation was considered by the Court of Appeals for the Fifth Circuit in a 1971 case emanating from Texas, involving natural gas producers who operated under a system not entirely dissimilar from health care regulation.[15]

Natural gas production is regulated in Texas to prevent excess extraction and resulting waste of resources. The allowable production for a particular well is set each month by a state regulatory agency in an effort to cause output to equal a reasonably anticipated demand and to allow each producer to enjoy its fair share of that market demand. The regulatory commission in this instance determined future demand through forecasts filed by all producers, then applied a pro rata formula to determine the allowable production for each.

One group of producers charged, however, that another group had subverted the pro rata formula by filing false forecasts in order to reduce allowable production. The defendants sought immunity for their conduct, contending the First Amendment's protections applied and characterizing their conduct as influencing government in a legislative context. The court disagreed, however, and analogized the process as more similar to the licensing procedure in the trucking industry, which was characterized properly as adjudicatory.[16] The court defined the critical distinction as being between efforts to influence government policy-making decisions and mere efforts to affect the outcome of the application of those previously determined policies. In this instance, the regulatory commission already had reached all policy decisions and mere implementation of the formula was not a political process, the court said. It ruled that the effort to undermine the efficacy of the application of a rule for anticompetitive purposes deserved no immunity.

It may appear that if the gas case decision is taken as applicable to the certificate of need process, health care providers are well advised to expect little, if any, protection for their essentially apolitical activities involved in providing the competitive impact information necessary to permit the system to function.

The application of the general rule of *Trucking, Unlimited* to health care providers is hardly limited to the certificate of need process, however. Where, for example, providers use the administrative and judicial processes to prevent actual or potential competitors from receiving state licensing or corporate permits, or to impose the cloud of potential state disapproval of the operations of the competitor, the adjudicatory process may be similarly abused, the competitor may be denied free and open access to tribunals, and immunities may not protect such conduct.[17]

Numerous disputes have developed regarding the extent to which those who utilize adjudicatory bodies in efforts to prevent competition or eliminate competitors may depart from the argument of meritorious causes and still enjoy the shield (or even sword) of their First Amendment protections. Certainly it can be concluded that where those who seek anticompetitive results actually prevail before the adjudicatory bodies, they are within their rights in so doing. However, where arguments and actions are determined to be unmeritorious, more difficult questions arise, and different courts have offered varying answers.

One federal district court in Texas in a 1976 case said it was difficult to draw the line between the protected intent to influence the adjudicatory process and the unprotected intent to abuse this process to the disadvantage of a competitor. If, however, a party could demonstrate that others instituted litigation with the *purpose* of achieving an objective other than that appearing on the face of the lawsuit and that the defendants had committed acts directed at attaining that collateral objective (other than acts ordinarily incident to the use of the courts) then the defendants have gone beyond the limits of the applicable immunities.[18]

A federal court in Missouri in 1977 similarly emphasized that the important distinction in such an action was between the institution of sham proceedings, which certainly was not protected by First Amendment immunities, and the use of sham and spurious legal arguments during valid proceedings. Where there was no pattern of baseless proceedings, mere sham legal arguments would not have caused the loss of First Amendment protections, the court ruled.[19]

More recently, courts have abandoned the previously expressed requirement of showing a pattern of multiple, baseless lawsuits or regulatory proceedings and have ruled that a demonstration that parties filed even a single sham and baseless lawsuit with the intention of interfering directly with the business of a competitor was sufficient to go beyond the protection of the First Amendment and result in a violation of the antitrust laws.[20]

An additional area of dispute over the presence of this immunity for the benefit of health care providers has concerned the question of what type of adjudicatory body actually qualifies as "governmental." Certainly Professional Standards Review Organizations, being bodies created by federal statute to serve regulatory functions, should qualify as governmental adjudicatory bodies when they operate in a decision-making mode. When the decision-making function has been delegated to the hospital, the immunity also should apply, although the question becomes an ever closer one and may be applied in an ever narrower fashion.

Medical staff review committees also frequently perform adjudicative type functions involving the conduct or acceptability of other physicians. Where state law confers a quasi-governmental status upon such committees, the usual immunities may be available. However, where state law does not confer some type of governmental status specifically on such committees, immunity for anticompetitive influences over the committees may not be available. This issue was addressed, for example, by a federal appellate court in a 1978 Florida case.[21] The court considered a state law that conferred evidentiary protections on the records of the medical staff review committee in question. The state law, however, did not give the review committee the power to issue final decisions on the conduct of physicians being reviewed. Rather, the committee's decisions were in the form of recommendations to another state agency. The role of the committee thus was not a governmental one, the court ruled, and no immunity was available for those who pursued an anticompetitive scheme through influencing the committee.[22]

Provider Efforts To Influence Governmental Purchases

A third capacity in which health care providers have both the motive and the opportunity to attempt to influence officials' decisions arises in dealing with governmental agencies in their proprietary capacities as purchasers of services such as health care services for government employees and for subsidized programs such as Medicare and Medicaid. Here, again, some providers may be inclined toward less than ethical practices, such as deception and misrepresentation in convincing government procurement or reimbursement agents to deal only with selected providers, to the anticompetitive exclusion of rivals.

If taken literally, the Noerr-Pennington immunity might appear at first to protect abusive publicity campaigns and misrepresentations directed toward influencing government purchasing decisions. In fact, at least one court did take the immunity just this literally and held that activities pursued to influence public procurement officials to specify products so narrowly as to eliminate those of competitors were constitutionally protected.[23] No appeal was taken from that case, however, so the decision was not tested by an appellate court.

The more recent and more rational view, however, has been that there exists no reason to confer an antitrust immunity on sellers of goods and services who deal with governmental purchasers they would not enjoy in dealing with private purchasers. The Noerr-Pennington rationale—that permitting every interest to be heard will produce tolerable political results from politicians fully informed of the opinions and desires of the political constituency—simply has no place in the theoretically apolitical world of government purchasing decisions. Here, on the contrary, the government is acting essentially in the same capacity as would a private purchaser and ordinarily desires the best products for its price, just as would a private buyer.[24]

Consequently, when dealing with government as a purchaser of health care services, no immunity whatsoever from the ordinary application of the antitrust laws should be anticipated from this fact alone. The First Amendment will not provide the same degree of protection to purely commercial activity as it does to attempts at political persuasion, and immunity for efforts to influence public officials in the adoption or enforcement of laws will not extend to efforts to sell services, or presumably influence individual reimbursement decisions.

This in itself does not mean, however, that efforts to influence legislative decisions on purchasing or reimbursement policies, or efforts to persuade administrative tribunals to issue desired reimbursement findings (such as the Provider Reimbursement Review Board) as always will not enjoy the immunities. This means only that anticompetitive efforts to influence government purchases and payments outside of legislative or adjudicatory contexts and only within government's proprietary functions most likely will receive no special immunity.

ANTITRUST IMMUNITY UNDER HEALTH PLANNING AND OTHER LAWS

The tension between the antitrust statutes, requiring free and open competition, and health planning laws, encouraging the elimination of competition through shared services and other means to reduce costs, is apparent immediately. The scope of government regulation, with at least the ostensible purpose of containing cost increases, seemingly is forever increasing, and pressures to respond in new and sometimes creative ways can come from various stimuli.

Hospitals and other institutional providers, for example, may be required by state law to obtain a certificate of need before beginning an expansion program, or even prior to replacing equipment or remodeling quarters. The process of receiving this required certificate, however, may involve numerous more subtle pressures to assure the desired outcome. As providers find that battling before the local Health Systems Agency (HSA) in order to defeat rival applications for certificates of need tends only to defeat the interests of all involved, they may find incentives toward cooperating voluntarily and privately in their own informal health planning processes. Similarly, they may do such informal health planning at the direct request of the local HSA, or perhaps even under its direction and subject to the threat of adverse recommendations to the state health planning agency should the hospitals fail in such concerted planning activities.

Effective health planning mechanisms seeking to eliminate the duplication of services and reduce excess capacity may gravitate naturally toward functions such as:

- the division of markets in order to create local monopolies and thus eliminate duplicate services

- the creation and exchange of long-range plans for new services so that each provider may know what other providers intend to do and structure its own plans accordingly
- the consolidation of services among various providers so that all may share a single service rather than compete for the provision of this service
- the abandonment of projects that appear to be potentially competitive with those of other providers

Similarly, industry groups have encountered incentives for creating nongovernmental cost containment mechanisms, such as the well known "voluntary effort" instigated by the challenge of a United States Congressman.

Response to pressures for cost containment thus may require or at least encourage anticompetitive behavior of a most overt nature. Health planning often is treated as synonymous with eliminating competition, or at least establishing mechanisms to avoid excessive competition. Standard antitrust analysis teaches that agreements among competitors to divide markets or to eliminate potential competition restrain trade and violate the Sherman Act. A similar conclusion would be reached on agreements to set prices. Consequently, providers must confront the question of the extent to which the antitrust laws potentially inhibit and restrict conduct that might be characterized either as cost containment and health planning or as market division and conspiracy to restrain trade.

In addressing the contradictory regulatory requirements (such as antitrust enforcement versus cost containment through health planning), the courts applying antitrust principles have developed a sometimes vague and complex set of rules whereby the apparently opposing requirements may be determined to be, in fact, to some extent reconcilable and to that extent concurrently enforceable. To the extent that the competing regulatory schemes are irreconcilably repugnant, however, one set of standards must be applied at the expense of the other. As far as the federal antitrust laws thus are irreparably repugnant to a federal regulatory (such as health planning) scheme, the antitrust laws will be deemed repealed by implication to the minimum extent necessary to allow the regulatory scheme to operate. (This is known as the doctrine of "implied repeal" and often is explained in connection with a similar and sometimes synonymous doctrine known as "exclusive jurisdiction," which essentially means that the administrative agency enjoys jurisdiction to the exclusion of the courts.)

Where federal antitrust laws conflict with a state regulatory scheme, the antitrust implications are somewhat more complex. Generally, however, where the anticompetitive state regulatory system is consistent with other federal laws, the state doctrine will provide immunity to providers compelled by the state, in its capacity as a sovereign entity, to undertake anticompetitive conduct. Additional and ever more complex issues are raised where no federal laws specifically demonstrate that Congress ever envisioned the anticompetitive state regulatory scheme; where the anticompetitive conduct was compelled by a governmental or quasi-governmental agency other than the state itself; or where the challenged conduct was perhaps instigated, but not directly compelled, by the state regulatory system.

Therefore a discussion of the rules of law that may provide antitrust immunity to health care providers participating in anticompetitive cost containment activities is appropriate, along with an exploration of probable applications of these rules and potential methods for increasing the chances of successfully invoking the immunity doctrines.

Implied Repeal and Agency Jurisdiction

With respect to efforts toward reconciling competing demands of antitrust policy and specific industry regulations, the Supreme Court consistently has articulated a relatively simple and dependable general rule or "guiding principle" to the effect that repeal of the antitrust laws will be regarded as implied only if necessary to make the specific industry regulation work, and even then only to the minimum extent necessary.[25] The application of this guiding principle to determine whether specific conduct is protected by such an implied repeal in the context of a specific industry regulatory scheme, however, is far from simple or clear. In fact, some trial courts have lamented that, notwithstanding the Supreme Court's decisions on the subject, definitive functional guidelines are not always discernible.[26]

In the effort to articulate functional standards, some courts have set forth lists of tests that may be applied to the challenged conduct, as illustrated by a four-part test established in 1977 by one federal court:[27]

1. Does the subject matter of the antitrust suit fall within the scope of a pervasive regulatory scheme established by Congress? This test essentially involves the question of whether the regulatory scheme is directed particularly at the type of conduct challenged in the subsequent antitrust suit.
2. Does the regulatory agency actively exercise its authority and subject the challenged conduct to meaningful review and regulation? This test demonstrates that mere agency approval will not create an antitrust immunity. However, such approval often is critical to a finding of implied immunity and certainly helpful toward that end.
3. Is the agency, under its regulatory scheme, authorized to consider antitrust concerns of the type that will arise in a judicial proceeding under the antitrust laws? In this test, it is significant that the agency is given power to remedy a potential antitrust violation by withholding its approval or requiring appropriate modification of prospective conduct.
4. Would the application of the antitrust laws to the regulated party subject it to conflicting or differing standards of conduct? In view of the unfairness

of subjecting a single entity to conflicting standards, an exemption may be implied to preserve the integrity of the regulatory system and protect a party from conflicting judicial judgments.

Even the efforts of the courts to abstract functional, practical tests for determining the applicability of the implied repeal doctrine, as exemplified by these examples, certainly have not succeeded in establishing benchmarks that are either entirely consistent among the various courts or entirely practical and determinative in analyzing prospective conduct. Consequently, it is instructive to consider the experience of a particular regulated industry that frequently has suffered the scrutiny of both the antitrust laws and a restrictive regulatory scheme: the securities industry.

This industry is subject to one of the more pervasive regulatory schemes in this country's legal and economic framework and has been the subject of a series of Supreme Court decisions on the relationship between the principles and functions of this regulatory scheme and the antitrust laws. For example, the securities regulations require self-policing of the conduct of brokers and dealers through the stock exchanges. This self-policing function was addressed by the Supreme Court in *Silver v. New York Stock Exchange*.[28] The questioned conduct involved the Stock Exchange's ordering its member firms to remove private direct phone lines with a nonmember firm under an exchange rule that did not provide for notice or a hearing on the decision to order the disconnection. The regulatory scheme also did not provide for review of individual enforcement decisions of this nature by the Securities and Exchange Commission (SEC), although the statute did grant the SEC the power to disapprove the stock exchange's rules, such as the one that required this disconnection.

The court held that the conduct could be challenged as a group boycott of the nonmember firms and that no implied repeal of the antitrust laws was effectuated by the regulatory scheme. In essence, it ruled that the enforcement of the antitrust laws was not repugnant to the operation of the regulatory scheme with respect to this type of conduct, notwithstanding a statutory grant of general powers to the exchange to regulate relationships between members and nonmembers. The SEC was not empowered to review the potentially undesirable anticompetitive effects of individual instances of self-policing within the exchange and there was no other method of assuring that some attention would be given to the public interest in competition, the court declared.

A different result ensued, however, from the Supreme Court's consideration of two subsequent efforts to apply antitrust scrutiny in the securities industry. In *Gordon v. New York Stock Exchange*[29] and *United States v. National Association of Securities Dealers, Inc.*[30] (which opinions were issued on the same day in 1975), the court determined that the regulation of the securities industry did serve to impliedly repeal the antitrust laws to some extent. In *Gordon,* the court said the system of fixed commission rates then in effect,[31] in which the exchanges set rates under the supervision of the SEC, was immune from antitrust attack. The court explained the critical distinctions between the *Gordon* and *Silver* cases, as:[32]

1. Although the exchanges set rates in the first instance, the action was studied actively and supervised by the SEC, and Congress clearly and directly had delegated this authority to the SEC.
2. The SEC could require alteration or supplementation of practices for the protection of investors.
3. In practice, all rate changes actually had been brought to the SEC's attention, and it always had taken an active role in reviewing proposed changes.
4. To permit operation of the antitrust laws in setting commission rates would interfere unduly with the operation of the Securities Exchange Act, particularly as antitrust scrutiny could cause the stock exchanges to face inconsistent requirements of SEC review and antitrust scrutiny. The court gave particular attention to the difference between, on the one hand, the SEC's mandate to supervise rate setting in view not only of competition but also of considering the economic health of investors, the exchanges, and the securities industry, and on the other hand the antitrust laws that, to the contrary, would require consideration of rate setting in view only of competition.

Similarly, in the *National Association of Securities Dealers* (NASD) case, the court declared that the antitrust laws were repealed by implication to the extent necessary to permit the SEC to exercise its statutory duties to regulate the conduct of the mutual fund industry. In this instance, the court conducted a detailed examination of the history of that industry and the reasons for the adoption of federal laws that eliminated some forms of price competition, inhibited the resale of mutual funds through a secondary securities market, and conferred on the SEC the authority to oversee agreements among brokers and dealers in mutual funds, restricting the terms upon which these securities could be traded.

The court concluded that, because of some of the unique problems of the industry, Congress had made a judgment that certain restrictions on competition were necessary and had vested in the SEC the final authority to determine whether and to what extent such restrictions should be tolerated, considering the interests of the holders of outstanding securities.

The *Silver, Gordon,* and *NASD* cases thus demonstrate the extremes of potential results, i.e., conduct either entirely without immunity and subject to antitrust attack in the courts, or conduct entirely immunized, with members of the industry subject only to the regulatory jurisdiction of the agency directly responsible for supervising that conduct.

A case involving the somewhat similar regulation of commodities exchanges demonstrates a form of intermediate result sometimes reached in order to defer the consideration of antitrust issues. In *Ricci v. Chicago Mercantile Exchange*,[33] a member of the defendant commodities exchange charged that the exchange and certain other members had conspired to restrain his business by transferring his exchange membership to another person without notice or a hearing. The plaintiff contended that this conduct constituted a violation of the antitrust laws and of the rules of the exchange itself.

The court explained that Congress had established the Commodity Exchange Commission specifically to determine whether exchange rules had been violated, and that this determination would be useful to a court later attempting to decide whether antitrust laws had been violated. Consequently, the court held that an antitrust action must await the prior administrative resolution of the validity of the challenged conduct within the regulatory scheme of that industry, and expressed optimism that the administrative process itself would help explain the scope, meaning, and significance of the administrative rules. Although the agency could not itself effect a repeal of the antitrust laws, its own decision-making process could assist the court in deciding to what extent this industry regulation produced an implied repeal of the laws.[34]

The problems that have beset the investment industries may help illustrate results that might ensue from agency regulation of particular conduct. Together with the tests abstracted by courts that have attempted to set forth step-by-step methods for determining the extent of any asserted implied repeal of the antitrust laws, these examples offer some help in predicting the application of the doctrine in the health care industry. These experiences, however, certainly do not offer the type of definitive tests that might be relied upon with confidence in structuring provider conduct.

Federal legislation establishing health planning policies and procedures is markedly different from the regulation of entry into, and growth within, any other industry. Public Law 93-641 (the National Health Planning and Resources Development Act of 1974) continues to be the substantive federal health planning law, notwithstanding repeated attempts to modify and supplement it. However, it is only partially self-implementing, calling instead upon the states to carry out significant portions of the nation's overall health planning policies. Although it is safe to conclude that the conduct of providers in permitting and assisting the health planning agencies in executing the functions required of them by P.L. 93-641 is immunized from antitrust attack under the implied repeal doctrine, this conclusion must be reached in further recognition of the presumption against implied repeal and the availability of this form of immunity only to the minimum extent necessary to allow the regulatory program to work.

As the implied repeal doctrine relates to federal, not state, law, it is the federal aspects of health planning that are directly relevant to the present evaluation.

Relatively few aspects of health planning, however, are conducted directly pursuant to federal law. P.L. 93-641 does establish some federal functions for health systems agencies that it directs be established, but it reserves more of the active and germane aspects of health planning to health systems agencies under state programs and to state health planning agencies themselves. The federal law does, however, provide guidelines and goals for health planning, as well as a structure for agency action, a list of functions for health systems agencies, and a mechanism for establishing criteria for health planning decisions.

Health planning thus is a joint effort, carried out primarily by state agencies but under general guidelines established by federal law for states that choose to comply with the voluntary federal standards. While some states may choose not to comply with all federal standards, individual noncomplying state health planning programs nevertheless may be in compliance with many aspects of the federal law, and almost certainly will be in conformance with the general federal goals and guidelines.

The proper analysis of the availability of antitrust immunities for providers engaging in some form of health planning or related cost containment efforts, therefore, requires consideration of the types of immunities state programs may confer, whether operating directly under federal goals and guidelines or under a state's more original efforts to contain or restrict health care costs and to influence the distribution of health care resources.

State Action

Although an individual state may not repeal or even contravene the federal laws and policies in the Sherman Act and other federal antitrust laws, it may establish and enforce a program to regulate a particular industry, with anticompetitive purposes and effects, where the program is not directly inconsistent with federal law.[35] The Supreme Court ruled explicitly in 1943 that the federal antitrust laws were not intended to apply to the conduct of a sovereign state or state officials in executing its valid regulatory policies.[36]

The case generally credited with creating, or first specifically recognizing, the "state action" exemption from the antitrust laws involved a California agricultural program that restricted competition among raisin growers and maintained prices in the marketing of raisins.[37] The program had been adopted by the state to help prevent overproduction and excessive competition in the marketing of agricultural products, with the objective of stabilizing prices in that industry. One raisin producer sued the California Director of Agriculture and other state officials, contending that the California program violated both the Sherman Act and the Federal Agricultural Marketing Agreement Act. The Supreme Court decided that the marketing program could be assumed to violate the Sherman Act if undertaken by private persons and that Congress could, in the exercise of its power to regulate interstate commerce, prohibit a state from maintaining such a program.

The court held, however, that the defendants in this context were immune from the antitrust laws because there was no indication that the Sherman Act was intended to restrain a state in regulating a particular industry where the regulation was not contrary to a superior federal law. Consequently, the state action exemption, often referred to as the *Parker v. Brown* doctrine after this case, provides that federal antitrust laws do not proscribe a state or its agents and officials from carrying out a valid state regulatory program. Notably, the court added that the state scheme was not contrary to federal policy, as federal law on agricultural marketing actually envisioned such programs. The court added the caveats that this was not a situation where the state had attempted simply to authorize others to violate the Sherman Act, an authorization that would confer no immunity, and there was no suggestion that the state or its agents had joined with others to participate in a private agreement to restrain trade. Presumably, these latter circumstances could change the outcome of the analysis.

For some time after *Parker v. Brown,* the state action immunity was applied on a relatively broad scope. More recently, however, significant questions have developed regarding the doctrine's applicability to the conduct of private parties or lesser governmental agencies, as courts have applied this exemption on an ever narrower basis.

The further explication and continued narrowing of the state action exemption has occurred through a series of Supreme Court cases, commencing in 1975 with *Goldfarb v. Virginia State Bar.*[38] In that case, the court addressed issues relating to the legality of the conduct of the Virginia State Bar Association and a county bar association in publishing an attorney fee schedule that created a rigid floor price below which local attorneys could not go in establishing their own individual fees. A client who was forced to pay the established price for legal services sued, contending that this activity constituted price fixing. The bar associations replied that the conduct did not violate the Sherman Act as: (1) there was a lack of impact on interstate commerce, (2) there was a total exemption from the antitrust laws for conduct within the learned professions, and (3) the state action exemption immunized the activities of the bar associations.

The court's opinion is of major significance to those engaged in conduct regulated by the states, as well as all persons in a learned profession (including those in the health care industry). The court ruled that neither the jurisdictional requirement of demonstrating an impact upon interstate commerce nor the contention that the conduct of a learned profession was exempt from the antitrust laws would protect the bar associations. The services were provided in connection with interstate transactions, and there simply was no exemption for the learned professions from the antitrust laws. The court then discussed the inapplicability of the state action exemption in these circumstances:

1. The states do have a compelling interest in the practice of professions within their boundaries and have a broad power to establish licensing standards and to regulate the practice of professions, and a state may determine validly that some forms of ordinary business competition may be demoralizing to the ethical standards of a profession.[39] The court thus validated general state regulatory practices over professions as not being inherently contrary to federal policy.

2. In determining whether particular anticompetitive conduct was immunized by the state action exemption, however, the court said the threshold inquiry was whether that conduct was required by the state acting as sovereign. In this instance, Virginia had not actually required the challenged conduct of either the state or county bar associations and had not required either bar association to issue fee schedules or establish floor prices. Even if the bar associations' activities were "prompted" by the objectives of the state's ethical codes, such prompting will not establish a state action exemption, the court found. Actual state *compulsion* of the conduct is a requisite, it said. As the state bar had joined with the county bar in establishing enforcement mechanisms to assure compliance with the county bar's fee schedules, the court ruled, both associations were in violation of the Sherman Act.

Consequently, *Goldfarb* established the principle that parties other than the sovereign state itself would not be immunized by the state action doctrine unless their conduct actually was compelled (not merely prompted) by the state acting in its capacity as sovereign. The court later applied this rule to the State Bar of Arizona,[40] which had issued an ethical rule prohibiting attorneys from advertising their fees. Although the court found that the rule violated the First Amendment guarantee of freedom of speech, the state action doctrine prevented the rule from constituting an antitrust violation.

The critical distinctions between the Arizona situation and *Goldfarb* were that the Arizona Supreme Court itself had issued the challenged rule, pursuant to a delegation of this responsibility from the State of Arizona acting as sovereign, and that the state actively reexamined these rules through its Supreme Court, under the state's important interest in regulating the legal profession. The state's direct involvement in compelling the challenged conduct thus conferred an antitrust immunity.

The possibility that what appears simplistically to be state compulsion to perpetrate particular conduct may in fact have been contrived by a private party for its own benefit was considered by the Supreme Court in 1976 in *Cantor v. Detroit Edison Company*.[41] The court held that no state action immunity was conferred by such contrived compulsion. The defendant electric utility in this case was subject to the pervasive regulation of the Michigan Public Service Commission, which was responsible for setting the rates the utility could charge for electricity. In 1916 the utility had caused the commission to endorse a practice in which the company provided its electricity customers with free light bulbs, the cost being absorbed in the charges for power. Thereafter, the commission required the utility to continue providing light bulbs without charge and said the company could not alter this practice without an express change in regulations by the commission. More than 50 years after this rule was adopted and enforced by the commission, a retailer of light bulbs (his business being hindered by the utility's free distribution system) sued Detroit Edison, contending that the program constituted the tying of electricity sales to light bulb distribution, contrary to the Sherman Act. The utility contended that the program was compelled by the state regulatory agency, thus conferring a state action exemption.

The court found that the state action exemption did not apply in these circumstances and that the utility could be held liable for its conduct, with the following rationales for this decision:[42]

1. The questioned program was the product of a decision in which both the utility and the regulatory commission participated. The option to have or not to have the program, in a long-run sense, was primarily that of the utility company, even though a departure from the program would require the commission's approval.
2. Although there might be circumstances in which the state's participation was so dominant that it would be unfair to hold the private party responsible for the conduct, this was not such a circumstance.
3. The state had no affirmative regulatory policy on the distribution of light bulbs, as opposed to electricity. This essentially was an unregulated market, so the program was not necessary to the functioning of the state's regulatory policy. Even if there were a possibility of conflict between that policy and the antitrust laws, the standards to be applied in resolving the potential conflict must be at least as strict as those applied to federal regulatory legislation (the implied repeal doctrine).
4. Mere state authorization, approval, encouragement, or participation in restrictive private conduct conferred no antitrust immunity. Where the private party exerted a sufficient degree of freedom of choice in its conduct, it would be held responsible. Consequently, this form of contrived compulsion did not confer immunity.[43]

The state action exemption being thus limited in its protection of the conduct of private parties, the Supreme Court in a 1978 case considered the availability of the doctrine to protect the conduct of municipalities, which some observers and courts previously had assumed enjoyed essentially the same immunity as that of the state under which the municipalities were created. The Supreme Court, however, found to the contrary, emphasizing at length the presumption against exclusions from the antitrust laws and the differences in the federal deference extended to government agencies in a sovereign state from that extended to the state itself. The court concluded that the state action doctrine would exempt from antitrust prosecution the conduct of a state's subdivision only where the challenged conduct was executed pursuant to state policy to displace competition with regulation or monopoly public service.[44]

Health Care Applications

Notwithstanding the vast potential number of applications of the implied repeal and state action doctrines to health care providers, there have been relatively few actual published decisions in the area. The following three examples, while not purporting to be exhaustive of the experiences of providers on the subject, should serve to illustrate at least partially the treatment that might be expected in future situations.

In *Traveler's Insurance Company v. Blue Cross of Western Pennsylvania,*[45] a federal trial court ruled in 1969 that the alleged conduct of the Blue Cross Association, in using its dominant position in the health insurance market to require preferential service contracts from hospitals with which it did business, was not immunized by the state action exemption. The court reached this result in spite of the pervasive regulation of the insurance industry by the Commonwealth of Pennsylvania that included regulation of rates charged to subscribers, rates of payments to hospitals, acquisition costs of new subscribers, reserves to be maintained, and all contracts between Blue Cross and hospitals. The court concluded that Blue Cross was not itself the creature of the state and the state had not specifically extended authority to engage in monopolistic practices.

Although the plaintiff was a rival insurance company and the hospitals involved in the agreements with Blue Cross were considered to be coerced and unwilling participants rather than active coconspirators with Blue Cross, the potential exposure of the hospitals in such a situation is apparent. For example, if the plaintiff insurance company in this case had alleged that the hospitals had conspired and agreed with Blue Cross to engage in reciprocal favors as part of a scheme intended to injure the competitive position of the plaintiff company, there would appear to be no reason to expect the pervasive state regulation of the contracts between hospitals and Blue Cross to confer any immunity for the challenged conduct. Similarly, there would seem to be no health planning policies served by such conduct, so no immunity should be forthcoming from that regulatory arena either.

In *City of Fairfax v. Fairfax Hospital Association,*[46] a county hospital association and other defendants sought to assert the state action defense on behalf of local government agencies, similar to the assertion of that defense as addressed by the Supreme Court in the *Louisiana Power and Light* case, and with similar results. In this instance, the plaintiff city, along with a group of physicians, sued a county hospital association and a government industrial development authority to prevent the development agency from purchasing a private hospital and leasing it to the county hospital association. The proposed purchase and lease would have given the county association control of the only two hospital facilities in that area. The plaintiffs specifically charged monopolization and that the contract constituted an unreasonable restraint of trade. A federal appellate court said, in part, that whether the challenged purchase by the industrial development authority and lease to the county hospital association constituted exempt state action was a question of fact to be determined at trial.

The facts that were not sufficient in themselves to constitute state action were essentially as follows:

The county hospital association had leased the land and its first facility from the county. The lease required the association to advise the county of its actions, to submit to the county its proposed budget before adoption, and to submit important contracts for comment before their execution. The county, however, was not shown to have a veto power, amendment power, or any other coercive power of control. The court stated that the facts did not prove that the Commonwealth of Virginia had compelled the county hospital association to do anything or that the state in the strictest sense regulated the hospital.

The state may well have been merely a landlord, financier, and reviewer of budgets and contracts, the court said. Furthermore, any commands from the county hospital association to the industrial development authority came from the county, the court held, and this lesser governmental agency did not automatically confer the exemption that would go with actual state action. Relying on *Goldfarb*, the court stated:

> The mere fact that a body is a state agency for some limited purposes does not make it an antitrust shield that allows it to foster anticompetitive practices.

Although the *Fairfax* case does not literally relate to health planning pursuant to P.L. 93-641 or any state certificate of need statute, the analogies are apparent. This was, in essence, an informal type of local health planning through provider consolidation. The state program, however, did not coercively mandate the consolidation of these hospitals and services. Even though P.L. 93-641 was in effect at the time of the *Fairfax* decision, and its overt encouragement of joint planning among hospitals to avoid proliferation of duplicated services could have been considered, the conduct in question was not mandated by state or federal law, nor would the disallowance of this informal type of health planning through provider consolidation be irreparably repugnant to the operation of the formal state and federal health planning programs.

The availability of the state action exemption to immunize the allegedly anti-competitive conduct of a state health care official was considered by an appellate court in *Feminist Women's Health Center, Inc. v. Mohammad*.[47] In this case (other aspects of which are discussed in other chapters), an abortion clinic charged that certain persons, including the executive director of the State Board of Medical Examiners, had conspired to boycott the clinic, among other forms of anticompetitive conduct. The executive director contended that the State Medical Practice Act conferred upon him a state action immunity, as the act was intended to protect the public against the improper practice of medicine and against professional irresponsibility, and that his challenged conduct was intended to improve the quality of medical care in the state.

The court, however, decided that this state position would not immunize the conduct of the director if the conduct was undertaken in his private or personal capacity rather than as a part of his job. Consequently, the court held, the exemption question became a factual one, depending upon whether the director perpetrated the challenged conduct as part of his job in executing the regulatory policies of the state as opposed to merely executing anticompetitive conduct beyond or outside of those regulatory policies.

Similar disputes can be anticipated in the context of health planning as state and local health planning officials enjoy antitrust immunity for conduct appropriate in carrying out state and federal health planning programs, but may not anticipate immunity where the conduct is executed for their personal gain or outside of the scope of any valid formal health planning programs.[48]

The extent of the immunities and exemptions conferred upon those functioning in health planning processes, whether in public or private capacities, should be a matter of increasing concern as more providers and health planning officials experiment with new methods of planning, and as more providers become disappointed by denials of expansion projects or approvals of rivals' projects. The general rules of implied repeal and the state action exemption are, of course, of some help in predicting the probable resolution of disputes in this field, and it can be stated with certainty that conduct involving federal health planning programs and valid state programs will be immunized at least to the minimum extent necessary to permit the programs to function. The following more specific situations may help illustrate considerations in this area:

1. Although one state supreme court (North Carolina) in 1973 held a state's certificate of need type law to be in excess of the constitutional powers of the state's legislature,[49] that result preceded the federal adoption of P.L. 93-641 and is unlikely to constitute a recurring problem. In fact, the specific mandates of the federal health planning law, encouraging the states to

adopt conforming laws in order to implement the federal policy, clearly will serve to bring conforming state laws within even the narrowest interpretation of the *Parker v. Brown* doctrine, as Congress has directed specifically that unrestricted competition is not now perceived to be the optimal method of allocating resources and responding to consumer needs in the health care industry. Consistent with this conclusion, one federal trial court concluded early in 1979 that the health planning laws were instituted specifically to displace competition in this industry, and therefore dismissed an action against an HSA and certain providers.[50]

2. The activities of a state health planning agency in Indiana in encouraging three private hospitals to submit a joint application to fill community bed needs, and the conduct of the hospitals in meeting, agreeing, and submitting such a proposal at the request of the agency, have been held to be consistent with the Medicare Section 1122 program and not, in the circumstances of that case, to constitute agency favoritism of the three joint applicants to the disadvantage of a fourth local hospital that suffered the denial of its individual planning application.[51]

Although this latter case did not include any overt recognition of potential antitrust issues, an appropriate hypothetical analysis of the facts of that case under the antitrust rules discussed above might proceed as follows:

1. The state health plan and health planning review functions were undertaken in connection with, and as necessary to implement, the federal Medicare program specifically under the requirements of Section 1122. The state health planning agency was acting directly as an agent of the Secretary of Health, Education, and Welfare, and not simply as an agent of the state itself. Consequently, the implied repeal doctrine was applicable to resolve any tensions between the administration of this federal regulatory scheme (notwithstanding the designation of a state agency to conduct these federal functions).

2. Acting under the federal regulatory program, the state agency had prepared a health plan, calculating bed need within the area in question and concluding that 172 additional beds were required.

3. Pursuant to the federal program, the agency had solicited individual project applications to fill the community bed need.

4. No single hospital submitted an individual proposal that fulfilled community need, and no combination of individual proposals met this need.

5. The planning agency decided a joint proposal was the only way the health planning program could actually fulfill community need, and therefore was the least restrictive anticompetitive conduct necessary to allow the federal regulatory program to work.

6. A significant regulatory review safeguard was offered because the joint proposal was meaningless unless the planning agency approved the application. The review process would allow for the receipt of adverse contentions by the hospital not participating in the joint application. If the private conduct went no further than to jointly solicit agency approval, First Amendment immunities might also be available.

Although this analysis indicates one method of finding the joint application process to be immune from antitrust concerns (in addition to potential First Amendment immunities as described in the previous section), additional facts or alternative circumstances indicate the importance of the following types of considerations when joint planning activities occur in the future.

1. Is the private joint application process truly the only alternative available to the planning agency? If the agency could fill community needs through individual hospital applications or by working with individual hospitals, this might indicate that the private agreement of the providers is not essential to the operation of the regulatory program.
2. Are individual providers being boycotted purposely by the joint planning activities? An attempt to use joint planning and agency approval to eliminate a competitor would help indicate that the particular planning activity was unlikely to be compelled by federal or state law or reasonably necessary to implement the health planning program. There is no indication in the federal law that health planning is intended to serve as a sword with which private participants jointly may eliminate rivals.
3. Is the planning agency acting as a coconspirator with some providers to disadvantage rival providers? *Parker v. Brown* distinguished situations where a regulatory agency itself was a member of an anticompetitive conspiracy beyond the scope of the regulatory process, presumably indicating the inapplicability of otherwise available exemptions.
4. Is the planning agency acting in the capacity of an agent of the federal government, as opposed to the state government? Where the planning agency is operating as a state agent, pursuant to state law, the additional questions raised by *Goldfarb, Cantor,* and *City of Lafayette* become significant. In such a situation, the parties must consider whether the state law under which the agency is operating with respect to specific conduct somehow is inconsistent with federal policy, whether the planning agency has delegated the functions of state health planning and is carrying out the delegated activities of the state in its sovereign capacity, and whether the conduct in issue has been compelled by the state, as opposed to merely prompted or encouraged.

5. Does the planning agency have the authority to consider the anticompetitive effects of the conduct in issue? Does it in fact do so? Would the application of the antitrust laws to the conduct in question effectively nullify the agency's regulatory powers? Courts generally have indicated that where competition and monopoly actually are considered by the regulatory agency, the courts at least will defer to such agency consideration first.[52] Where the subsequent judicial application of the antitrust laws would jeopardize the agency's authority to carry out its regulatory functions, the agency jurisdiction may be exclusive.[53]

6. Is the challenged conduct merely made possible by a regulatory program, rather than an integral aspect of that program? The resulting nonimmunity of such a situation was explained in 1977 by a federal trial court in Oregon where regulatory approval of the acquisition of certain assets by a dominant company put that company in a position to disadvantage its competitors later. The court said, in essence, that although the acquisition itself might be exempted from antitrust attack by virtue of the regulatory approval, subsequent conduct merely made possible by the acquisition was not exempt.[54]

In sum, formal health planning processes may be expected to confer immunities for conduct that health planning agencies find necessary to carry out their actual statutory duties, as well as duties compelled by valid regulations, where the resulting compulsion is not somehow contrived by providers or directly contrary to federal law. The health planning statutes, however, nowhere indicate an intent to validate overtly predatory (intended to eliminate rivals) private conduct, such as group boycotts or private price fixing at levels intolerable to rivals.

Providers may improve their chances of immunizing health planning conduct by making a complete record of all competitive impact considerations during hearings before health systems agencies and state health planning agencies. These agencies will assist in this effort by receiving and thoroughly considering opposing arguments based on anticompetitive factors. In addition, private and public participants in health planning should be careful that while working together toward common goals of appropriate provision of health care services they do not become coconspirators in predatory conduct or other anticompetitive schemes.[55]

Two significant areas of recent concern regarding the antitrust ramifications of cost containment programs are the potentially anticompetitive impact of state rate review programs and the conduct of the "voluntary effort," whereby hospital associations privately have established programs and guidelines toward cost containment.

State-conducted rate setting or rate review programs provide an additional form of regulatory activity, presumably in the interest of cost containment, beyond the specific scope of P.L. 93-641 or other federal law. The federal conclusion of the undesirability of unrestrained competition in the health care sector, however, certainly prevents any serious contention that a state rate review program necessarily is contrary to federal policy. The validity of, and exemption conferred by, any such system is essentially an individual question, depending upon the details of the particular program. The Antitrust Division of the Department of Justice has reviewed at least one such program (Wisconsin's) and found it unobjectionable from the perspective of federal antitrust law, although the division explicitly reserved the right to challenge particular conduct under the program later.[56]

As with other regulatory programs, private parties participating in this form of price fixing can anticipate exemption from antitrust liability where their conduct is only that compelled by the state or an agency to which the state has specifically delegated this function.[57] The potential for adverse consequences, as with any regulatory scheme, includes the possibility that private parties eventually will control the price-fixing functions of the program, with state participation reduced to mere authorization, encouragement, or acquiescence, or that private participants may take advantage of opportunities created by the regulatory process to conspire independently on matters beyond the scope of the agency regulation.[58]

The voluntary effort of various hospital associations to cause their members to reduce the rate of cost increases, contrary to the type of mandatory rate review considered above, presents an almost classic situation of governmental prompting and encouragement without compulsion or active supervision and, consequently, without the extension of any antitrust immunities. The very notion of voluntary compliance with industry-established mechanisms for containing costs, in the absence of governmental regulation, is contrary to the basic tenets of the implied repeal and state action doctrines. However, it certainly is possible that a self-imposed industry effort to control spiralling costs through collective efforts to operate in an efficient manner and individual actions to avoid unnecessary duplication of services could be conducted without violating the antitrust laws. No special exemptions or immunities, however, should be anticipated.

Numerous other health planning and related cost containment regulatory activities may be expected to raise questions regarding the potential implied repeal and state action immunities. Although each instance of challenged conduct must be considered and analyzed individually, in each case the critical analysis should be similar to the various analyses here.

NOTES
1. 365 U.S. 127, 81 S.Ct. 523 (1961).
2. *Id.*, at 365 U.S. 144, 81 S.Ct. 533.
3. 381 U.S. 657, 85 S.Ct. 1585 (1965).

4. *Id.*, at 381 U.S. 670, 85 S.Ct. 1593.

5. *Id.*, at 381 U.S. 671, 85 S.Ct. 1594.

6. *See, e.g., Franchise Realty, Interstate Corporation v. San Francisco Local Joint Executive Board of Culinary Workers*, 542 F.2d 1076 (9th Cir. 1976); *Charlotte Telecasters, Inc. v. Jefferson-Pilot Corp.*, 1977—1 Trade Cases (CCH) ¶ 61,304 (W.D.N.C. 1974).

7. *Subscription Television, Inc. v. S. Calif. Theater Owners Ass'n*, 576 F.2d 230 (9th Cir. 1978).

8. *Mark Aero, Inc. v. TWA, Inc.*, 580 F.2d 288 (8th Cir. 1978).

9. *Metro Cable Co. v. CATV of Rockford, Inc.*, 516 F.2d 220 (7th Cir. 1975).

10. *Hospital Bldg. Co. v. Trustees of Rex Hosp.*, 425 U.S. 738, 96 S.Ct. 1848 (1976).

11. *Duke and Co., Inc. v. Foerster*, 521 F.2d 1277 (3rd Cir. 1975).

12. Compare, *Harman v. Valley Nat'l Bank of Ariz.*, 339 F.2d 564 (9th Cir. 1964), to *Sun Valley Disposal Co. v. Silver State Disposal Co.*, 420 F.2d 341 (9th Cir. 1969); notwithstanding the 9th Circuit's apparent retreat from its position in the *Harman* case, the Supreme Court appears to have approved this decision through reference in *California Motor Transport Co. v. Trucking, Unlimited*, 404 U.S. 508, 513, 92 S.Ct. 609, 613 (1972).

13. *California Motor Transport Co. v. Trucking, Unlimited, supra*, note 12.

14. The Supreme Court next applied the rule of *Trucking, Unlimited* in *Otter Tail Power Co. v. United States*, 410 U.S. 366, 93 S.Ct. 1022 (1973), again holding that where the use of the courts to suppress competition takes the form of insubstantial claims, the use of the courts may be a sham, and the immunity is lost.

15. *Woods Exploration and Producing Co. v. Aluminum Co. of Am.*, 438 F.2d 1286 (5th Cir. 1971), *cert. denied* 404 U.S. 1047 (1972).

16. At the time of the *Woods* decision, the Supreme Court had not issued the *Trucking, Unlimited* opinion, but the 9th Circuit had done so, and it is this opinion to which the court referred in *Woods*.

17. *See, e.g., Health Corp. of America v. N.J. Dental Ass'n*, 1977—1 Trade Cases (CCH) ¶ 61,232 (D.N.J. 1977), where the plaintiff alleged that the defendants had instituted sham lawsuits and regulatory court proceedings and disseminated misleading information to induce dentists not to contract with the plaintiffs.

18. *Associated Radio Service Co. v. Page Airways, Inc.*, 414 F.Supp. 1088 (N.D. Tex. 1976).

19. *Central Bank of Clayton v. Clayton Bank*, 1977—1 Trade Cases (CCH) ¶ 61,422 (E.D. Mo. 1977).

20. *See, e.g., Cyborg Systems, Inc. v. Management Science of America, Inc.*, 1978—Trade Cases (CCH) ¶ 61,927 (N.D. Ill. 1978).

21. *Feminist Women's Health Center, Inc. v. Mohammad*, 586 F.2d 530 (5th Cir. 1978).

22. The defendants contended that the committee functioned in a legislative capacity. It would seem likely, however, that such committees frequently function in a manner more adjudicative than legislative in nature.

23. *United States v. Johns-Manville Corp.*, 259 F.Supp. 440 (E.D. Pa. 1966).

24. Some courts have indicated that where a government purchasing program demonstrates interests apart from buying products within a competitive system, then this additional factor should be considered in determining whether some sort of immunity is appropriately conferred. *See, George R. Whitten, Jr., Inc. v. Paddock Pool Builders, Inc.*, 424 F.2d 25, 32 (1st Cir. 1970).

25. *Gordon v. New York Stock Exchange*, 422 U.S. 659, 683, 95 S.Ct. 2598, 2612 (1975).

26. *See, e.g., United States v. CBS, Inc.*, 1977—1 Trade Cases (CCH) ¶ 61,327 (C.D. Cal. 1977).

27. *Id.*, at 71,134-5. *See also, Phonetele, Inc. v. AT&T*, 435 F. Supp. 207 (C.D. Cal. 1977), applying a similar four-part test.

28. 373 U.S. 341, 83 S.Ct. 1246 (1963).

29. 422 U.S. 659, 95 S.Ct. 2598 (1975), *supra,* note 25.

30. 422 U.S. 694, 95 S.Ct. 2427 (1975).

31. Fixed commissions have since been repealed in favor of competitive rates.

32. 422 U.S. 689, 95 S.Ct. 2615 (1975).

33. 409 U.S. 289, 93 S.Ct. 573 (1973).

34. The doctrine of primary jurisdiction was applied similarly by a federal trial court in *Macom Products Corp. v. AT&T,* 359 F.Supp. 973 (C.D. Cal. 1973). The court explained that the administrative proceedings could make significant contributions to the resolution of the antitrust lawsuit.

35. *See, e.g., Olsen v. Smith,* 195 U.S. 332, 25 S.Ct. 52 (1904).

36. *Parker v. Brown,* 317 U.S. 341, 63 S.Ct. 307 (1943).

37. *Id.*

38. 421 U.S. 773, 95 S.Ct. 2004 (1975).

39. *Id.,* at 792, 95 S.Ct. 2016.

40. *Bates v. State Bar of Arizona,* 97 S.Ct. 2691 (1977).

41. 28 U.S. 579, 96 S.Ct. 3110 (1976).

42. This decision was agreed upon among a plurality of the justices, and therefore it would be inappropriate to set forth the entirety of the opinion as that of the court. The various bases nevertheless may be valuable for guidance.

43. A similar result was reached by the 5th Circuit in *Litton Systems, Inc. v. Southwestern Bell Telephone Co.,* 539 F.2d 418 (1976), where the doctrine of primary jurisdiction was held to be inapplicable to private conduct in which each state regulatory board had routinely acquiesced.

44. *City of Lafayette, Louisiana v. Louisiana Power and Light Co.,* 435 U.S. 389, 98 S.Ct. 1123 (1978). (This is also a plurality opinion.)

45. 298 F.Supp. 1109 (W.D. Pa. 1969).

46. 562 F.2d 280 (4th Cir. 1977). Although this case was vacated by the Supreme Court (98 S.Ct. 1642 (1978)) and remanded for reconsideration in light of the initial court's decision in *City of Lafayette, supra* note 44, the opinion does not appear to be inconsistent with *Lafayette.*

47. *Supra,* note 21.

48. *See, e.g., Hospital Bldg. Co. v. Trustees of Rex Hosp., supra,* note 10, where a local health planning official was named as a defendant in an alleged conspiracy to improperly use the health planning process to prevent the construction of a new hospital.

49. *In re* certificate of need for Aston Park Hosp., Inc., 282 N.C. 542, 193 S.E.2d 729 (N.C. 1973).

50. *Huron Valley Hospital, Inc. v. City of Pontiac,* 1979—1 Trade Cases (CCH) ¶ 62,520. It should be noted that the specific federal policy of instituting health planning programs through state law removes this industry from some of the problems that have occurred in attempting to resolve conflicts between anticompetitive state laws and federal antitrust policy. For example, in *Schwegmann Bros. v. Calvert Distillers Corp.,* 341 U.S. 384; 71 S.Ct. 745 (1951), the Supreme Court ruled that a state resale price maintenance program was contrary to the policies of the Sherman Act and could not be enforced. Similarly, in *Rice v. ABC Appeals Board,* 21 Cal.3d 431, the California Supreme Court attributed constitutional dimensions to the policies of the Sherman Act and held that California's own liquor price maintenance program was contrary to that act and, therefore, invalid. Where federal and state regulatory policies specifically concur, however, as with the certificate of need programs of states that conform to federal law, this type of conflict should not arise. For states that choose to go demonstrably beyond or contrary to federal health planning programs, the issues still might need to be addressed.

51. *Lakeside Mercy Hosp., Inc. v. Indiana State Board of Health*, 421 F. Supp. 193 (N.D. Ind. 1976).

52. *See, e.g., Macom Products Corp., supra,* note 34.

53. *Hughes Tool Company v. TWA, Inc.*, 409 U.S. 363, 93 S.Ct. 647 (1973).

54. *Mt. Hood Stages, Inc. v. Greyhound Corp.*, 555 F.2d 687 (9th Cir. 1977).

55. Although Pub. L. 93-641 provides immunity for HSA officials insofar as their conduct is within the scope of their duties, it does not purport to provide immunity for conduct beyond the scope of their valid activities.

56. This was the program of the State of Wisconsin, described at 1978—1 Trade Cases (CCH) ¶ 62,000 at 74,277.

57. *See,* especially, the analysis of a potential rate review program by the Iowa Attorney General at 1978—1 Trade Cases (CCH) ¶ 62,000.

58. Potential antitrust exposure for conduct in connection with rate setting activities is discussed in *United States v. Southern Motor Carriers Rate Conference*, 1977—2 Trade Cases (CCH) ¶ 61,551 (N.D. Ga. 1977).

Chapter 4

Mergers, Acquisitions, and Affiliations

The economic tensions that confront health care providers, created by both free market and regulatory pressures, frequently develop incentives toward consolidations and affiliations. Regulatory pressures to reduce costs, for example, may generate incentives toward multiinstitutional arrangements of various natures. So, too, will the need to meet competition within the industry effectively as existing chains and group affiliations are perceived to hold advantages in competing in markets for additional facilities, physicians, and administrative staff. Efforts to gain the advantages of larger operations can take various levels of formality and severity, ranging from loosely organized shared service organizations to actual mergers of facilities or of parent corporations.

Examples of the results of pressures toward consolidation and affiliation include:

- the recent merger of the third and fourth largest hospital chains, creating the nation's largest chain organization, owning and managing 115 hospitals with 18,492 beds
- efforts by Catholic hospitals toward forming a network of 100 hospitals, with 17,800 beds, involving the pooling of assets into an umbrella corporation to provide shared services and management expertise[1]
- reported 29 percent rise in management contracts by multiunit hospital systems during 1978 in both proprietary and nonprofit hospital management organizations[2]
- mergers of local hospitals, with or without related mergers of their staffs[3]
- local joint ventures toward sharing services[4]
- affiliations and/or consolidations of hospitals and health maintenance organizations, or other purchasers of hospital services[5]

A related trend, though probably the result of quite different incentives, is the increasing emphasis on the formation of medical group practices through the consolidation or affiliation of physicians through various mechanisms.

Although many of these affiliations and consolidations may result in valuable economies or improved quality in the delivery of health care, whenever the number of independent market factors (here, health care providers) is reduced within some segment of the market, antitrust ramifications are present.

For analytical purposes, it is important to note that consolidations and affiliations can take different forms in both legal and business aspects. For example, a consolidation may be achieved through a statutory merger, an outright purchase of stock or assets, a joint venture through a pooling of assets, or the formation of a joint subsidiary. In addition, affiliations may be achieved through the formation of associations, federations, consortiums, or similar organizations. The market impact of a lease, a management contract, or even an exclusive contractual arrangement may be similar to an actual consolidation and therefore might be analyzed under similar legal principles. Each method of achieving the desired result may have distinct legal consequences in areas of taxation, corporate law, and government regulation, in addition to antitrust.

These options for consolidations and affiliations (hereafter referred to as consolidations) suggest one manner of legal analysis of the impact of consolidating. However, an additional level of analysis is required to account for the differences in the anticipated market impact, depending upon whether the consolidation is horizontal (involving competitors), vertical (ordinarily involving entities in a buyer-seller or analogous relationship), or conglomerate (involving entities that are not technically horizontal or vertical, but may be engaged in services or products complementary to each other).

As illustrated below, the market relationship of the parties generally is more consequential to the legality of the consolidation than is the technical form the linkup may take. Accordingly, the analysis of actual and hypothetical consolidations in this chapter generally will emphasize the relationships of the parties over the form of the affiliation.

THE APPLICABLE LAWS

The federal law most directly applicable to, and most specifically restrictive of, corporate consolidations is Section 7 of the Clayton Act. The basic restrictions in this section are:

> No corporation engaged in commerce shall acquire, directly or indirectly, the whole or any part of the stock or other share capital and no corporation subject to the jurisdiction of the Federal Trade Commission shall acquire the whole or any part of the assets of another corporation engaged also in commerce, where in any line of commerce in any section of the country, the effect of such acquisition may be substantially to lessen competition, or to tend to create a monopoly.

No corporation shall acquire, directly or indirectly, the whole or any part of the stock or other share capital and no corporation subject to the jurisdiction of the Federal Trade Commission shall acquire the whole or any part of the assets of one or more corporations engaged in commerce, where in any line of commerce in any section of the country, the effect of such acquisition, of such stocks or assets, or of the use of such stock by the voting or granting of proxies or otherwise, may be substantially to lessen competition, or to tend to create a monopoly.[6]

In essence, Section 7 of the Clayton Act prohibits a corporation in interstate commerce from acquiring the stock or assets of another corporation where the effect may be to reduce competition or to tend to create a monopoly. For all of its restrictive applications, however, the exceptions to these restrictions often are more interesting than the restrictions themselves.

First, it is apparent immediately that Section 7 applies only to acquisitions of corporations by corporations. Consequently, where either the acquiring or the acquired entity is a partnership or unincorporated association, the statute does not apply.

Second, where the acquisition is through the purchase of assets, as opposed to a purchase of stock, the acquiring corporation must be subject to the jurisdiction of the Federal Trade Commission. Of peculiar importance in the health care industry is the statutory exclusion from FTC jurisdiction for corporations that are organized to carry on business neither for their own profit nor for the profit of their members.[7] Consequently, where a not-for-profit corporation (such as a hospital or chain of hospitals) acquires the assets of another corporation, Section 7 is arguably inapplicable if its literal terms are enforced. Conversely, however, if that same not-for-profit corporation acquired the stock or other share capital, rather than the assets, of the acquired company, and if the other jurisdictional elements of Section 7 were met, then the statute would apply.[8]

Third, Section 7 provides statutory exclusions for purchases of stock to be held for investment only when the stock is not used in voting or otherwise to help reduce competition.

Perhaps the most important jurisdictional requirement for the application of Section 7 in the context of the health care industry is that both the acquiring and the acquired corporations be "engaged in commerce." This requirement not only is semantically distinct from the Sherman Act's jurisdictional requirement that the challenged conduct have a "substantial effect" upon interstate commerce, but the Clayton Act requirement has been interpreted much more narrowly by the courts.

Thus, in *United States v. American Building Maintenance Industries,*[9] the Supreme Court held that Section 7 of the Clayton Act could not be applied to the acquisition of two local janitorial service corporations by one large intrastate (operating entirely within one state) janitorial service corporation. The court explained in detail that the "engaged in commerce" standard in the Clayton Act was different from the "affecting commerce" standard of the Sherman Act. Even where the acquiring corporation admittedly was engaged in commerce by virtue of its multifaceted interstate activities, the court said the acquired corporation here did not perform services outside the one state in which it operated, and the mere fact that these corporations purchased within the state supplies that had been manufactured outside the state did not cause the corporations to be "engaged in commerce."

Similarly, local health care providers might contend that their services are provided entirely intrastate. The mere fact that supplies were produced in other states, if analogized to the *American Building* situation, need not cause the provider to be engaged in commerce. If, however, substantial quantities of products are purchased directly in interstate commerce by the provider facility, the situation might be different from *American Building*. (That case is helpful because it specifically explains that Section 7 is not applicable to acquisitions of partnership assets or the assets of other unincorporated enterprises.[10])

In spite of the other limitations on the application of Section 7, the courts consistently have afforded a very broad definition of the phrase "acquire, directly or indirectly, the whole or any part of the stock . . . or any part of the assets . . . " The result of this broad interpretation is that the section can reach virtually any form of transfer of legal rights and privileges. For example, in *United States v. Columbia Pictures Corporation*,[11] a producer and distributor of films for television entered into a 14-year exclusive license with another producer and distributor for the exhibition of films. The court found that this license right constituted an asset of the licensor and consequently the licensee had acquired a part of the assets of the licensor, thus bringing the transaction under Section 7. The following language of the court, explaining the breadth of the reach of Section 7, provides useful analogies for the health care field:

> As used here, the words "acquire" and "assets" are not terms of art or technical legal language. [Footnote omitted.] In the context of this statute, they are generic, imprecise terms encompassing a broad spectrum of transactions whereby the acquiring person may accomplish the acquisition by means of purchase, assignment, lease, license, or otherwise. The test is pragmatic. The final answer is not in the dictionary.
>
> The statute imposes no specific method of acquisition. It is primarily concerned with the end result of a transfer of a sufficient part of the bundle of legal rights and privileges from the transferring person to the acquiring person to give the transfer economic significance and the proscribed adverse "effect."[12]

Consequently, it is apparent that institutions achieving joint ownership, control, or similar results may be subjected to the scrutiny of Section 7 notwithstanding the creativity with which they may structure the transaction.

It is worth repeating that Section 7 does not prohibit corporate acquisitions in and of themselves, but only restricts such acquisitions where the effect may be to lessen competition substantially or to tend to create a monopoly in some line of commerce in some section of the country. Consequently, each Section 7 case will require an analysis of the appropriate line of commerce and the appropriate section of the country to determine the likely effect upon competition there.

Beyond the applications of Section 7 of the Clayton Act, and as is true in most other aspects of antitrust law, the FTC can challenge an acquisition or consolidation as an unfair method of competition under Section 5 of the Federal Trade Commission Act, including acquisitions involving unincorporated entities that do not fall under Section 7 of the Clayton Act. Although Section 5 of the FTC act is much broader than Section 7 of the Clayton Act, the courts have determined that where an acquisition would be likely to violate Section 7 of the Clayton Act, it necessarily would be likely to violate Section 5 of the Federal Trade Commission Act.[13] How much broader the application of Section 5 of the FTC act might be, however, remains speculative.

In addition to the potential application of those two sections, Sections 1 and 2 of the Sherman Act remain valuable mechanisms to challenge consolidations and affiliations. Where an acquisition (no matter how broadly that term is used) may be characterized as a contract or combination in restraint of trade, or where such an acquisition creates a monopoly or may be characterized as an attempt to create a monopoly, then the Sherman Act becomes applicable, and the restrictive jurisdictional requirements of the Clayton Act become unimportant.

The potential application of the Sherman Act to challenge acquisitions of any sort may be particularly important in the health care industry, where facilities may well be found to impact upon interstate commerce even though they are not engaged in commerce. Furthermore, the Sherman Act imposes no requirement that the entities involved be formally incorporated. It should be noted, however, that the plaintiff must expect to incur the burden of proving a more substantial restraint of trade under Sherman Act tests than under Section 7 of the Clayton Act, although the extent of the divergence between the two statutes cannot be quantified.[14]

In at least one merger case, however, the Supreme Court relied upon an analysis taken from cases brought under Section 7 of the Clayton Act in order to find the challenged merger illegal under Section 1 of the Sherman Act.[15] Consequently, it may appear that while the explicit tests available under Section 1 of the Sherman Act require a higher standard of restraint of trade in order to find an illegality, a challenge to a merger will always be a challenge to a merger, and courts may be expected to blur somewhat the diverging standards in different statutes under which a merger may be challenged.

In addition to the statutory standards, the U.S. Department of Justice has issued relatively detailed guidelines on the types of situations in which it expects to challenge mergers. Although these guidelines do not have the force or effect of law, they frequently are afforded substantial respect by the courts and should not be ignored by the parties to a prospective consolidation. These guidelines will be considered in detail in connection with the different structural types of consolidations discussed below.

HORIZONTAL CONSOLIDATION IN THE HEALTH CARE INDUSTRY

The best known recent consolidation of major health care providers is the acquisition of American Medicorp (the third largest hospital chain) by Humana (the fourth largest), creating the largest hospital group in the country. The acquisition was accomplished by Humana's public tender offer for the shares of American Medicorp. The tender offer, which was contested by the management of American Medicorp, generated several judicial decisions, one of which is particularly useful in this analysis.[16]

American Medicorp (Medicorp) brought suit to prevent Humana's purchase of its shares through the tender offer, contending in part that if successful, this would constitute an acquisition in violation of Section 7 of the Clayton Act and Sections 1 and 2 of the Sherman Act. Medicorp requested that the court issue a preliminary injunction (an extraordinary remedy whereby a party may be enjoined from certain conduct prior to the final trial of the action) to prohibit Humana from making the tender offer.

The court's analysis, in determining the probability that the proposed acquisition would lessen competition substantially in some line of commerce in some section of the country or would otherwise constitute an unreasonable restraint of trade or create a monopoly, offers insights into the mechanisms and theories through which acquisitions in the health care industry may be challenged.

Initially, Medicorp contended that hospitals actually competed in two lines of commerce: (1) construction, management, acquisition, and replacement; (2) the providing of medical services to patients and of medical facilities to doctors.

Both Medicorp and Humana operated on a national scale, and Medicorp contended that the analysis of the proposed acquisition must account for the fact that only proprietary chains that operated on such a national scale were similar competitors, and purely local facilities did not compete on this somewhat rarefied scale unique to the leading chain organizations. By isolating national proprietary chains, Medicorp was able to contend that the acquisition would leave the combined company with a market share of 29.5 percent, and could demonstrate that this was a concentrated type of market in that the top eight firms controlled 84.2 percent of the hospital beds in the market consisting solely of national proprietary chains.

As for the second line of commerce—the delivery of hospital services to patients and physicians—the two companies could not be considered direct competitors on a national scale. Rather, hospital services by their nature are provided in a localized area and consequently it is necessary to consider the impact of the acquisition in various local geographic areas. Medicorp contended that the proposed consolidation would result in a lessening of competition in three local geographic markets.

The court extensively analyzed each of the contentions that led Medicorp to conclude that there existed a line of commerce in the hospital industry other than the providing of medical services and facilities for the practice of medicine. As to the contention that other aspects of the industry could form a separate line of commerce, the court said in essence:

- The development of new hospitals does not constitute a line of commerce. Development opportunities simply are not commercially distinct from the market for the product or service the company seeks to expand by the consolidation. The need for proprietary chains to expand and develop, the sale of these development services to community groups, and the need for the community support for development services—created in part by the need for community support in order to obtain certificates of need to permit the desired development—do not cause the building of new proprietary hospitals to constitute a separate line of commerce, distinct from the provision of medical services.
- There is no separate line of commerce composed of the management of hospitals. In this instance, Medicorp and Humana were not competing for management contracts.
- There is no separate line of commerce consisting of the acquisition of hospitals distinct from the provision of medical services through hospitals. The demonstrated fact that Medicorp had been an active acquirer of hospitals did not serve to demonstrate the existence of a new line of commerce.
- There is no separate line of commerce consisting of replacement activities (the substitution of new facilities for outmoded ones and the expansion of services and/or beds in so doing) distinct from the providing of medical services through hospitals. A hospital does not engage in significant competition in replacing itself other than the competition it may encounter during the regulatory process from those seeking to cause the denial of approvals for the replacements. Even if there were a separate market for such replacement activities, however, this line of commerce would have to be analyzed in the context of the local geographic market, not of a national market, as competition would occur on a local rather than a national scale.
- There is no distinct submarket consisting of proprietary chains. Even

though such chains may compete for investment capital in a manner very different from a nonprofit hospital's investment capital-raising activities, this distinction is not relevant in determining the existence of a separate line of commerce. Medicorp did not demonstrate that a proprietary chain offered such a unique cluster of services that it was significantly insulated from competition from local or multiinstitutional nonprofit competitors.

The court also said it disagreed with Medicorp's suggested definition of the appropriate geographic market for analytical purposes. Medicorp, as noted, had singled out proprietary competitors on a national scale. The court held, however, that each local health service area must be considered a relevant section of the country in determining the probability that the proposed acquisition would lessen competition substantially within each such health service area.

Although the combined corporation formed by the merger of Humana and Medicorp would control only 1.7 percent of the licensed hospital beds in the United States, it would control substantially greater percentages in particular local geographic markets. Medicorp therefore contended that the proposed merger would result in Humana's owning or operating 16.9 percent of the licensed beds in one county in Florida, 27.5 percent in a county in Kentucky, and 100 percent in a town in West Virginia.

The court further found, however, that those county and town geographic delineations lacked a sufficient evidentiary base to conclude that they were appropriate geographic markets for analytical purposes and that Medicorp had not demonstrated that its hospitals in the two counties actually competed for patients or doctors with those operated by Humana. Although Medicorp had demonstrated a likelihood that competition would be lessened substantially in the West Virginia town, it had not shown the irreparable injury that is necessary to obtain relief before trial.

The Medicorp case is interesting particularly for the court's simplifying the definition of the relevant product market in hospital merger situations, *i.e.*, the operation and management of short-term acute care community hospitals. The court also offered a simplified definition of the relevant geographic market in such situations, *i.e.*, each health service area is a relevant geographic market in which a party challenging a proposed merger must demonstrate the probability of a substantial lessening of competition. (The relevance of the health service area as a geographic market might be challenged in particular instances, however, where for example the hospital is located at the edge of the health service area or offers unique services that in practice compete with those of more distant hospitals.)

The Medicorp case also is interesting for the court's total omission of any possibility that the hospitals might have been providing specialized services that did not actually compete with each other. (For example, an acute care hospital that specializes in orthopedic services would not seem to compete directly with a neighboring acute care hospital that specializes in the treatment of cardiac patients.) Rather, the court defined the relevant product market as simply the operation and management of short-term acute care community hospitals.

CONSOLIDATION AT THE LOCAL LEVEL

Although the Clayton Act's jurisdictional requirement that each of the corporations involved be "engaged in commerce" should have been met easily by each of the national hospital chains in *Medicorp v. Humana*, this may not be true of a merger of two local hospitals where no multistate parent corporations are involved. However, such a local consolidation may be challenged under Sections 1 and 2 of the Sherman Act. Just such a situation was presented in *City of Fairfax v. Fairfax Hospital Association.*[17] This involved the acquisition of one of two hospitals in a Virginia county by the other hospital. The consequence of this consolidation was that all hospital services in that county then were controlled by a single agency. The consolidation was challenged by a group of physicians and a city within the county. They charged that the acquisition constituted a contract and combination in restraint of trade, and the creation of a monopoly, violating Sections 1 and 2 of the Sherman Act.

Although the decision did not involve the actual trial and determination of the case (the only issue at this level was whether there were sufficient triable facts to allow the plaintiff to proceed to trial), the court did find that the challenged conduct had sufficient impact upon interstate commerce to bring the transaction within the Sherman Act and that the plaintiffs were persons who might be able to prove that the consolidation had adverse effects upon their direct pecuniary interests and, therefore, were entitled to bring the action to protect those interests. (The defendants' contention that the transaction was insulated by the state action doctrine was discussed in Chapter 3.)

The significance of this case is in demonstrating the applicability of Sections 1 and 2 of the Sherman Act to a simple consolidation of local hospitals and the possibility that local physicians and other persons may consider themselves financially injured by such a consolidation and thus be inclined toward bringing an action either to prevent the consolidation or to recover damages to compensate for their losses.

Aside from the obvious types of horizontal consolidations represented by the mergers of neighboring national chain general acute care hospitals, other types of horizontal consolidation may be expected to raise sensitivities in the health care industry. For example, where neighboring hospitals form a shared service organization to consolidate particular services, a horizontal consolidation may be achieved. In the long run, this type of consolidation may be less damaging than an actual merger of hospitals, as the former might be reversed more easily.

Nevertheless, in the short run, or as long as the joint venture or shared service organization continues to operate, the impact on the market for the particular services that are consolidated is the same as that achieved by an actual merger of the facilities.

In essence, consumers who formerly relied upon, and perhaps benefited from, the availability of multiple providers of services now are presented with a reduced number of providers—perhaps only one. Similarly, suppliers who previously could sell, to multiple purchasers may be forced now to deal with a single purchaser. In the context of the health care industry, the results of these types of horizontal consolidations may range from the enhancement of both the quality and the economy of the providing of medical services, on the positive side, to the elimination of the medical practice of particular physicians, on the negative side.

An example of the diversity of perceptions of the consequences of hospital mergers can be seen by comparing the experience described by the director of medical affairs at two Denver hospitals concerning the merger of their medical staffs with the dissatisfaction of a physician who lost his radiology practice when two neighboring hospitals in another state merged.[18] Dr. William Robinson, the Denver medical affairs director, describes a very favorable result through the merger of the medical staffs, obviously including substantial cooperation on the part of the two hospitals. The merger led to the closing of the pediatrics unit at one hospital and of the obstetrical unit at the other. Dr. Robinson indicates no particular dissatisfaction from the physicians affected and attests to the increased economy and quality of the consolidated units.

Conversely, however, when the two hospitals in Clarksburg, West Virginia, merged, eliminating one of two radiology departments in that town, the radiologist who lost his departmental contract was aggrieved. Rather than oppose the merger itself, he challenged the exclusive arrangement between the consolidated institution and the radiologist who contracted to operate the department. The court dismissed this Sherman Act challenge to the exclusive departmental contract, but it seems entirely possible that physicians disadvantaged in this manner in the future may choose to challenge the consolidation itself as a combination constituting an unreasonable restraint of trade that damages the business or property of the disadvantaged physician.

JUSTICE GUIDELINES ON HORIZONTAL MERGERS

Because of the sensitivity to horizontal consolidations in general, and the need for standards to help guide corporate planning, the courts and the Department of Justice have offered statements under the general test in Section 7 of the Clayton Act on classifications of horizontal mergers that may be particularly likely to substantially lessen competition in a market area. (Although these standards are not applicable directly to Sherman Act challenges to consolidations, the experience of *The First National Bank and Trust Company of Lexington*[19] indicates the general relevance of the Clayton Act, at least during a preliminary analysis of a merger that may be subjected only to Sherman Act scrutiny.)

The most precise standards for challenges to horizontal mergers are those offered by the Department of Justice. It should be reiterated that these guidelines do not form a legal standard. However, they do indicate the areas in which the department would expect to challenge a merger, and they have been afforded some respect by the courts. The department states its enforcement policy on horizontal mergers:

> In enforcing Section 7 against horizontal mergers, the Department accords primary significance to the size of the market share held by both the acquiring and the acquired firms. ("Acquiring firm" and "acquired firm" are used herein, in the case of horizontal mergers, simply as convenient designations of the firm with the larger market share and the firm with the smaller share, respectively, and do not refer to the legal form of the merger transaction.) The larger the market share held by the acquired firm, the more likely it is that the firm has been a substantial competitive influence in the market or that concentration in the market will be significantly increased. The larger the market share held by the acquiring firm, the more likely it is that an acquisition will move it toward, or further entrench it in, a position of dominance or of shared market power. Accordingly, the standards most often applied by the Department in determining whether to challenge horizontal mergers can be stated in terms of the sizes of the merging firms' market share.

***

5. Market Highly Concentrated.

In a market in which the shares of the four largest firms amount to approximately 75% or more, the Department will ordinarily challenge mergers between firms accounting for, approximately, the following percentages of the markets:

Acquiring Firm	**Acquired Firm**
4%	4% or more
10%	2% or more
15% or more	1% or more

(Percentages not shown in the above table should be interpolated proportionately to the percentages that are shown.)

6. Market Less Highly Concentrated.

In a market in which the shares of the four largest firms amount to less than approximately 75% the Department will ordinarily challenge mergers between firms accounting for, approximately, the following percentages of the market:

Acquiring Firm	**Acquired Firm**
5%	5% or more
10%	4% or more
15%	3% or more
20%	2% or more
25% or more	1% or more

(Percentages not shown in the above table should be interpolated proportionately to the percentages that are shown.)

7. Market With Trend Toward Concentration.

The Department applies an additional, stricter standard in determining whether to challenge mergers occurring in any market, not wholly unconcentrated, in which there is a significant trend toward increased concentration. Such a trend is considered to be present when the aggregate market share of any grouping of the largest firms in the market from the two largest to the eight largest has increased by approximately 7% or more of the market over a period of time extending from any base year 5-10 years prior to the merger (excluding any year in which some abnormal fluctuation in market shares occurred) up to the time of the merger. The Department will ordinarily challenge any acquisition, by any firm in a grouping of such largest firms showing the requisite increase in market share, of any firm whose market share amounts to approximately 2% or more.

8. Non-Market Share Standards.

Although in enforcing Section 7 against horizontal mergers the Department attaches primary importance to the market shares of the merging firms, achievement of the purposes of Section 7 occasionally requires the Department to challenge mergers which would not be challenged under the market share standards of Paragraphs 5, 6, and 7. The following are the two most common instances of this kind in which a challenge by the Department can ordinarily be anticipated:

(a) acquisition of a competitor which is a particularly 'disturbing,' 'disruptive,' or otherwise unusually competitive factor in the market; and

(b) a merger involving a substantial firm and a firm which, despite an insubstantial market share, possesses an unusual competitive potential or has an asset that confers an unusual competitive advantage (for example, the acquisition by a leading firm of a newcomer having a patent on a significantly improved product or production process).

There may also be certain horizontal mergers between makers of distinct products regarded as in the same line of commerce for reasons expressed . . . where some modification in the minimum market shares subject to challenge may be appropriate to reflect the imperfect substitutability of the two products.

It is apparent immediately that the department might expect to challenge what could be characterized as a rather ordinary hospital merger in that virtually any one is likely to involve facilities that hold market shares in excess of the standards cited, and local hospital markets are likely to be relatively concentrated by department standards.

STANDARDS SET BY THE COURTS

Although the standards set by the courts in determining which mergers might be presumed to substantially lessen competition, constitute unreasonable restraints of trade, or tend to create a monopoly, may be less precise than those of the Department of Justice, the judicial standards are not necessarily significantly more forgiving. For example, the proposed merger of two grocery store chains in Los Angeles was found by the Supreme Court to violate Section 7 of the Clayton Act because the chains, if joined, would account for 7.5 percent of groceries sold in that city.[20] The determination of illegality, however, could not be based solely upon a finding of this combined market share. Rather, the inquiry included the trend toward concentration in the industry, and the court found there was a trend toward a decrease in the number of competitive suppliers in this market.

In this context, the increasing of the market share of a consolidated supplier, at the expense of reducing the number of competitors in the market, becomes even more important. Furthermore, the court noted that both parties to the proposed merger had been expanding within the market and, therefore, could be viewed as very effective market factors whose elimination would be particularly detrimental to competition there.

Similarly, when the tenth largest beer brewer in the United States proposed to acquire the assets of the eighteenth largest brewer, forming a company that would hold 4.49 percent of the American market, the Supreme Court analyzed the acquisition with emphasis upon the trend toward concentration in that market. The court found that in various local submarkets, the combined company would enjoy a market share far in excess of the 4.49 percent national share. Emphasizing the trend toward concentration, the court determined that such an acquisition could violate Section 7 of the Clayton Act.[21] The courts also have emphasized nonmarket share factors where, for example, the merging companies are major competitive factors and the consolidation would significantly eliminate the competition between them.[22]

Although these rules are applicable in the development of a plaintiff's case in challenging an actual or prospective consolidation, certain—although generally limited—defenses do exist. In addition, as with other mergers, if the merging parties fulfill certain criteria, they may be required to give detailed advance notification to the Department of Justice and the FTC. (Both defenses and advance notification are discussed later.)

VERTICAL CONSOLIDATIONS

Vertical structure has been described as involving a buyer and seller relationship between the parties. Consumers, or buyers, of health care services probably are viewed most often as the patients themselves. The seller of health services generally is the health care facility or a physician. The consolidation of these types of entities seems unlikely to raise antitrust ramifications. There are, however, entities in the health care industry that may be tempted to seek consolidations or affiliations with their suppliers or their customers. For example, numerous health maintenance organizations (HMOs) are parties to contracts with acute care hospitals under which the HMOs purchase certain services, probably including predictable bed days of care, from the hospital. The HMO is spared the expense of establishing its own hospital facility, the hospital is given a guaranteed income for services purchased by the HMO, and the hospital and the HMO are in a vertical or buyer-seller relationship. The buyer-seller relationship also may take the form of the HMO's purchase of hospital services on a fee-for-service basis without the formality of a contractual arrangement.[23]

In the same manner, an employer that purchases HMO services for the benefit of its employees is in a buyer-seller, or vertical, relationship with the HMO. So, too, is a health insurance company that buys hospital or physician services in a vertical relationship with the parties from which it obtains those services.

In each of these examples of vertical relationships, so long as the parties remain independent of each other there is an opportunity for horizontal competition. For example, a second hospital may well decide to compete with the one that sells its services to the HMO in the first example. This not only affords the HMO the opportunity to extract the best possible bargain for hospital services, it also gives other hospitals the opportunity to sell their services to a substantial purchaser. Other HMOs also can compete for the purchase of hospital services, thus providing the hospital the opportunity to obtain a better bargain than if it were dealing with only a single purchaser.

Perhaps of even greater importance in the antitrust analysis of this hypothetical independent vertical relationship is the fact that as long as hospital services are available to the HMO in a locality, a new HMO may enter the market without encountering the barriers to entry that would be present if it were required to provide actual hospital facilities of its own. If no hospital facilities were available for purchase, however, the HMO would be forced to build facilities. Consequently, were the hospital and the HMO purchaser of hospital services to merge, the following types of market impact would become possible:

1. If the availability of hospital services to independent HMOs is reduced significantly by the merger, it may become that much more difficult for new HMOs to enter the market. Consequently, potential competition in the HMO portion of the market may be reduced, and actual competition may drop eventually.
2. If the available purchasers of services from other hospitals are reduced significantly by the merger, other hospitals may have to offer some sort of HMO services. A new hospital attempting to enter the market also would face this requirement. Although this might appear to be a stimulus toward the introduction of new competition in the HMO segment of the market, it also could work to reduce competition in the hospital segment.
3. If the hospital that previously provided services to the general purchaser continues to offer services, on a contract or fee-for-service basis, to an independent HMO after the merger, there may be an incentive to favor its own internal HMO at the expense of independent and competing HMOs. This may have the further tendency of reducing long-run competition in the HMO market.

Similar results may be hypothecated involving the consolidation of an HMO with an employer which purchases HMO services. In general, the problems are those of eliminating a buyer or seller from the market and thus reducing opportunities to sell to the eliminated buyer or purchase from the eliminated seller. Furthermore, where independent buyers and sellers are virtually eliminated from the market, potential new entrants to that market will be required to enter in a vertically integrated manner, as there will be a lack of nonintegrated outlets with which they may deal.

In spite of the problems vertical consolidations may create, in many instances they may benefit the ultimate consumer of the service or product—most likely the patient and/or the taxpayer, in the case of the health care industry. For example, vertical consolidations may eliminate major transaction costs and reduce quantitative uncertainties in providing health services. The consolidation of an HMO with a hospital eliminates the need for the HMO to build its own hospital facilities, thus helping to reduce possible local overcapacity, further reducing the cost of health care in general. It also has been suggested that consolidations with HMOs will reduce hospitals' collection problems, thus allowing the hospitals to more precisely predict revenues which would result in further cost savings.

JUSTICE GUIDELINES ON VERTICAL MERGERS

As with horizontal mergers, the Department of Justice has issued its own guidelines, constituting warnings of occasions on which the department anticipates challenging vertical mergers. These guidelines provide as follows:

***

12. Supplying Firm's Market.

In determining whether to challenge a vertical merger on the ground that it may significantly lessen existing or potential competition in the supplying firm's market, the Department attaches primary significance to (i) the market share of the supplying firm, (ii) the market share of the purchasing firm or firms, and (iii) the conditions of entry in the purchasing firm's market. Accordingly, the Department will ordinarily challenge a merger or series of mergers between a supplying firm, accounting for approximately 10% or more of the sales in its market, and one or more purchasing firms, accounting *in toto* for approximately 6% or more of the total purchases in the market, unless it clearly appears that there are no significant barriers to entry into the business of the purchasing firm or firms.

13. Purchasing Firm's Market.

Although the standard of paragraph 12 is designed to identify vertical mergers having likely anticompetitive effects in the supplying firm's market, adherence by the Department to that standard will also normally result in challenges being made to most of the vertical mergers which may have adverse effects in the purchasing firm's market (*i.e.*, that market comprised of the purchasing firm and its competitors engaged in resale of the supplying firm's product or in the sale of a product whose manufacture requires the supplying firm's product) since adverse effects in the purchasing firm's market will normally occur only as the result of significant vertical mergers involving supplying firms with market shares in excess of 10%. There remain, however, some important situations in which vertical mergers which are not subject to challenge under paragraph 12 (ordinarily because the purchasing firm accounts for less than 6% of the purchases in the supplying firm's market) will nonetheless be challenged by the Department on the ground that they raise entry barriers in the purchasing firm's market, or disadvantage the purchasing firm's competitors, by conferring upon the purchasing firm a significant supply advantage over unintegrated or partly integrated existing competitors or over potential competitors . . . .

14. Non-Market Share Standards.

(a) Although in enforcing Section 7 against vertical mergers the Department attaches primary importance to the market shares of the merging firms and the conditions of entry in the relevant markets, achievement of the purposes of Section 7 occasionally requires the Department to challenge mergers which would not be challenged under the market share standards of paragraphs 12 and 13. Clearly the most common instances in which challenge by the Department can ordinarily be anticipated are acquisitions of suppliers or customers by major firms in an industry in which (i) there has been, or is developing, a significant trend toward vertical integration by merger such that the trend, if unchallenged, would probably raise barriers to entry or impose a competitive disadvantage on unintegrated or partly integrated firms, and (ii) it does not clearly appear that the particular acquisition will result in significant economies of production or distribution unrelated to advertising or other promotional economies.

(b) A less common special situation in which a challenge by the Department can ordinarily be anticipated is the acquisition by a firm of a customer or supplier for the purpose of increasing the difficulty of potential competitors in entering the market of either the acquiring or acquired firm, or for the purpose of putting competitors of either the acquiring or acquired firm at an unwarranted disadvantage.

Consequently, where a vertical consolidation involves a firm situated in the capacity of supplier and accounting for 20 percent or more of the sales in its particular market, and a firm situated as buyer and accounting for 6 percent or more of purchases in that market, a challenge to the merger might well be anticipated.

Standards of legality for vertical consolidation established by the courts predictably are less extensively articulated than are the Department of Justice guidelines, and are not so generalized, but nevertheless must be relied upon for guidance to the extent possible. A useful example of a judicial analysis of a vertical merger is *United States v. Sybron Corporation*.[24] This merger was between a manufacturer and a retailer of dental products. The vertical relationship was that of the manufacturer as the seller and the retailer as the purchaser. The court first determined that the merger involved three lines of commerce—the overall dental products market and two submarkets (dental equipment and sundries). The appropriate section of the country, for antitrust analysis purposes, was determined by the court to be the nation as a whole. Taking these product markets and the geographic market, the court considered the probable impact of the merger with respect to the following indicia of competitive factors:

1. The foreclosure of retail outlets to other manufacturers;
2. The probability that the merged retailer, if it did continue to market the products of other manufacturers, would favor the products of its own intracorporate manufacturer;
3. The creation of barriers to entry at both the retailing and manufacturing levels generated by the increased vertical integration in the industry;
4. The historical trend toward increasing integration in the industry;
5. The market shares of the merged companies and the concentration level of the industry, finding that the manufacturer represented respectively 18.1, 4.3, and 9.2 percent of the three lines of commerce evaluated and that the retailer represented 6.5 percent, 7.5 percent, and 8 percent of those lines of commerce.

Based upon this analysis, the court found that the merger violated Section 7 of the Clayton Act.

Although the *Sybron* case helps illustrate the individual factors that should be analyzed in predicting or considering the legality of a vertical consolidation, each industry and each market must be analyzed as to its own peculiar facts to determine whether the consolidation may lessen competition substantially, constitute a combination in restraint of trade, or create a monopoly.

CONGLOMERATE CONSOLIDATIONS

Consolidations that are neither horizontal (in that no direct competitors are involved) nor vertical (in that the parties are not in a buyer-seller relationship) generally are referred to as conglomerate. As with so many other areas in health care, the appropriate characterization of what is conglomerate as opposed to vertical or horizontal is complicated by the traditionally independent contractor relationship between hospitals and physicians, notwithstanding the functional necessity for each to be available to the other and the intervention of the doctor in the relationship between the hospital and the patient who is the actual consumer of the hospital's services.

For this analysis, however, and although doctors frequently may be recognized as the major determinants of the purchase of hospital services, the physician in the hospital is not considered to be in a vertical relationship if not the actual purchaser of the services. Similarly, even though hospital personnel frequently may be the determinants of patients' purchases of services of extended care facilities, the hospital is not the buyer and the relationship will not be considered vertical.

Consequently, conglomerate consolidations in the health care industry may involve parties that previously enjoyed very close (although neither horizontal nor vertical) relationships. For example, if a large medical group were to purchase a hospital, the acquisition might well be characterized as a conglomerate consolidation. If a hospital or its parent company were to buy a skilled nursing facility, it could be considered a conglomerate consolidation. For similar reasons, if a large medical group specializing in pediatrics were to merge with another medical group specializing in orthopedics, this could be a conglomerate consolidation. In each of these examples, although the parties were neither direct competitors nor purchasers and sellers with each other, the consolidation would allow the now unified company or group to offer an expanded range of services in the health care market.

A different type of market expansion can be accomplished through conglomerate consolidations of corporations that operate in the same service market but in different geographic areas. For example, if a hospital chain that operated only in the Eastern United States merged with one that operated only in the Western United States, the parties could not be characterized as actual competitors, nor would they be in a buyer-seller relationship. Consequently, this is a type of conglomerate merger.

Although conglomerate consolidations, by definition, do not involve the immediate loss of direct competitors in a market, nor in the type of vertical integration that in itself may reduce competition or competitive opportunities, courts and numerous commentators have expressed a variety of reasons for disallowing conglomerate consolidations that meet certain criteria. Particularly during times of high corporate merger activity, there seems to be a fear that eventually the American economy may be reduced to the activities of a small number of huge conglomerates. Although no single merger might be determined to substantially lessen competition in a line of commerce in a section of the country, dissatisfaction frequently is expressed on the general trend toward the consolidation of economic units into a smaller number of larger companies.[25]

Beyond the general dissatisfaction created by perceptions of increasing economic concentration, the specific dangers created by certain conglomerate consolidations have been set forth by courts and commentators and relied upon by courts in analyzing the probability that a particular conglomerate merger may lessen competition substantially. Generally, conglomerate mergers are perceived to be particularly likely to threaten an eventual reduction in competition in one or more of three situations:

1. If the merger eliminates a potential entrant into a particular line of commerce or section of the country, thus eliminating the possibility that at some future date competition would have been increased in that particular market
2. If the merger creates a danger of reciprocal buying between the merged companies, thus eliminating competitive opportunities or outlets for independent companies
3. If the merger is particularly likely to entrench the market position of one of the companies such as through a major infusion of funds from the other company, that might be used to help the recipient exclude other competitors or potential competitors from that market

JUSTICE GUIDELINES ON CONGLOMERATE MERGERS

As with horizontal and vertical mergers, the Department of Justice has issued its own guidelines, warning when it anticipates challenging conglomerate mergers. The relevant operating portions of those warnings provide as follows;

The Department will ordinarily challenge any merger between one of the most likely entrants into the market and:

(i) any firm with approximately 25% or more of the market;
(ii) one of the two largest firms in a market in which the shares of the two largest firms amount to approximately 50% or more;
(iii) one of the four largest firms in a market in which the shares of the eight largest firms amount to approximately 75% or more, provided the merging firm's share of the market amounts to approximately 10% or more; or
(iv) one of the eight largest firms in a market in which the shares of these firms amount to approximately 75% or more, provided

either (A) the merging firm's share of the market is not insubstantial and there are no more than one or two likely entrants into the market, or (B) the merging firm is a rapidly growing firm. . . .

19. Mergers Creating Danger of Reciprocal Buying.

(a) Since reciprocal buying (*i.e.*, favoring one's customer when making purchases of a product which is sold by the customer) is an economically unjustified business practice which confers a competitive advantage on the favored firm unrelated to the merits of its product, the Department will ordinarily challenge any merger which creates a significant danger of reciprocal buying. Unless it clearly appears that some special market factor makes remote the possibility that reciprocal buying behavior will actually occur, the Department considers that a significant danger of reciprocal buying is present whenever approximately 15% or more of the total purchases in a market in which one of the merging firms' ("the selling firm") sales are accounted for by firms which also make substantial sales in markets where the other merging firm ("the buying firm") is both a substantial buyer and a more substantial buyer than all or most of the competitors of the selling firm.

(b) The Department will also ordinarily challenge (i) any merger undertaken for the purpose of facilitating the creation of reciprocal buying arrangements and (ii) any merger creating the possibility of any substantial reciprocal buying where one (or both) of the merging firms has within the recent past, or the merged firm has after consummation of the merger, actually engaged in reciprocal buying, or attempted directly or indirectly to induce firms with which it deals to engage in reciprocal buying in the product markets in which the possibility of reciprocal buying has been created. . . .

20. Mergers Which Entrench Market Power; Other Conglomerate Mergers.

The Department will ordinarily investigate the possibility of anticompetitive consequences, and may in particular circumstances bring suit, where an acquisition of a leading firm in a relatively concentrated or rapidly concentrating market may serve to entrench or increase the market power of that firm or raise barriers to entry in that market. Examples of this type of merger include:

(i) a merger which produces a very large disparity in absolute size between the merged firm and the largest remaining firms in the relevant markets, . . .

(iii) a merger which may enhance the ability of the merged firm to increase product differentiation in the relevant markets. . . .

The aspects of conglomerate consolidation that seriously raise the sensitivities in the Department of Justice are similar to the factors that have been most emphasized by the courts. A useful example of judicial examination of conglomerate mergers is that of the Supreme Court in *Federal Trade Commission v. Proctor & Gamble Company*,[26] where the court analyzed the acquisition of the nation's leading bleach producer (Clorox) by the largest producer of household detergents and similar products, not including bleach (Proctor & Gamble). The court offered a detailed analysis of the size of the two companies and the size of competitive companies, and concluded that where an already dominant, although somewhat smaller, firm such as Clorox was acquired by a much larger firm, such as Proctor & Gamble, the result could have a chilling effect on the probability of other firms' choosing to compete with the Clorox product.

In essence, the court concluded that the mere size of Proctor & Gamble as a corporation would create a disincentive to smaller firms from entering or choosing to compete more vigorously in the bleach market. It ruled that in effect this was an entrenchment or a market enhancement tending to demonstrate that the acquisition of this bleach manufacturer by a large corporation not involved in the manufacture of that product still could substantially lessen competition in that market.

The court also analyzed the history of Proctor & Gamble as a corporation and determined that it was a particularly likely new entrant into the bleach market, even without the acquisition of Clorox. Consequently, the merger would serve to eliminate the potential entrant (Proctor & Gamble) from the bleach market. Because of these factors, the court concluded that the acquisition of Clorox by Proctor & Gamble violated Section 7 of the Clayton Act. (Other conglomerate cases that would demonstrate useful caveats sometimes analogous to the health care industry are considered under Defenses.)

Certain analogies to the dangers of conglomerate mergers noted by the courts and the Department of Justice may carry through to the health care industry. For example, where a large group of physicians acquires a hospital, the dangers of reciprocal dealing are apparent. The physicians have a greater incentive to send their patients to the hospital they have acquired, and the hospital may tend to favor the owner-physicians on matters such as the granting of exclusive departmental contracts and other staff privileges. However, if the structure or history of the particular market can be demonstrated to indicate the unlikelihood of such a consequence, then the prospect of reciprocal dealing need not weigh heavily against the acquisition. Similar considerations may be applied to the hypothetical consolidation of two large physician groups, each specializing in different areas.

Many facets of the health care industry, however, do not lend themselves to similar analogies regarding other dangers of conglomerate mergers. For example, the acquisition of a local hospital by a large chain that had not operated in a locality would not appear, on its face, to put that hospital at a substantial advantage over others in the area that did not enjoy the support of a national chain. Nor would this acquisition be likely to remove the national chain as a potential entrant from the local market, due to the usual regulatory factors inhibiting hospital entry. To the extent that either of these conclusions is not true, however, this type of conglomerate consolidation might be challenged on the ordinary bases applicable to other industries.

DEFENSES

Throughout the development of the antimerger laws and guidelines, certain factors have been relied upon repeatedly by defendants in various actions to help demonstrate that the proposed consolidations did not offend any applicable law. Some of the defenses might be classified appropriately and legally as failures in proof of the plaintiffs' case while others might be actual defenses available even where the plaintiff succeeds in demonstrating a *prima facie* violation. For discussion purposes, these points will be classified simply as defenses, particularly for foreseeable situations in the health care industry.

Jurisdictional Defenses

As noted, the most restrictive antimerger law, Section 7 of the Clayton Act, applies only to consolidations between corporations and, even then, only where both corporations actually are engaged in commerce. Where unincorporated entities are involved, or where the entities may affect commerce without actually being in the stream of commerce, the plaintiff will be required to rely upon statutes other than Section 7, possibly including state antitrust laws which may or may not be as restrictive of consolidation activities as is Section 7.

It thus is possible that where, for example, physicians' groups are not incorporated and are the subject of anticonsolidation attacks, Section 7 of the Clayton Act may not apply for both of the reasons cited. Similarly, it is entirely possible that a local hospital may not be engaged in commerce, even though its activities may affect commerce.

Nonprofit Institutions

Nonprofit hospitals are not subject to the jurisdiction of the Federal Trade Commission and will have a defense to an action brought by that agency. Similarly, nonprofit hospitals may have a defense on this basis to a challenge under

Section 7 of the Clayton Act where the consolidation is achieved by way of a purchase of assets rather than a purchase of stock or a statutory merger.

Economies Through Consolidation

Both the courts and the Department of Justice have been unreceptive to contentions that a particular consolidation, even though it might tend to reduce competition in a line of commerce, will result in such economies in the providing of services or products that the consumers will receive a net benefit in spite of the possible reduction of competition.

Thus, in each of the three types of mergers discussed above, the Department of Justice guidelines provide that the decision to challenge a merger will not be influenced by a demonstration of economies produced by the merger because (1) the department does not believe the mergers it challenges are the type most likely to result in economies; (2) the available economies generally can be achieved through internal expansion rather than consolidation with existing companies; and (3) it usually is extremely difficult to accurately establish and quantify any claimed economies.

Even more directly, the Supreme Court in *Proctor & Gamble* declared:

> Possible economies cannot be used as a defense to illegality. Congress was aware that some mergers which lessen competition may also result in economies but it struck the balance in favor of protecting competition.[27]

Although economies in providing services or products generated by the challenged consolidations appear to be a disfavored defense, this result of the merger should not be overlooked entirely. For example, where the merger is vertical and its effects on competition are unclear, a demonstration of economies resulting in reduced prices to the consumer still might help persuade a tribunal that the consolidation is unlikely to substantially lessen competition.

The judicial dissatisfaction with the defense of economies should be subject to further scrutiny in the context of the health care industry. This industry is criticized frequently for not being subject to the same economic pressures as other industries because of the prevalence of third-party payers, perceived unresponsiveness of physicians to their patients' expenses (a perception certainly subject to some scrutiny itself), and generally inadequate information on the part of consumers.

Statutory and regulatory preferences for the development of any systems, multiinstitutional or otherwise, that achieve cost reductions in health care services and thus reduce prices paid both by government and by private payers may create the sort of Congressional recognition of the value of savings necessary to overcome the Clayton Act's failure to recognize or provide for a defense of increased economies in spite of decreased competition. In fact, P.L. 93-641 specifically encourages efforts to achieve just this sort of economy in health care services, and this mandate may prevail in demonstrating the legality of multiinstitutional arrangements where Clayton or Sherman Act standards are not clearly violated. P.L. 93-641 also should create an implied repeal of antitrust laws inconsistent with the operation of the federal health planning law. The question then becomes to what extent the antimerger laws actually are repugnant to P.L. 93-641.

Countervailing Power

Where a particular line of commerce may be dominated by certain large companies, or even where those companies do not dominate a market, it might be contended that the consolidation of two smaller firms would allow them in their new unified and larger form to compete more effectively with the larger companies. The notion that competition in a market may be more effective among, for example, four large firms than it would be among three large companies and two smaller ones has been referred to as the concept of "countervailing power."

If properly analyzed, this argument in the defense of a challenged consolidation really is a contention that the merger will not be likely to lessen competition but actually will be likely to increase it. Consequently, where a consolidation power can be demonstrated to be necessary for effective competition in a market area, this showing would appear to rebut the contention that the merger is likely to lessen competition.

However, if countervailing power has been asserted as necessary not to increase competition in a market but to allow local entities to compete more effectively in other geographic areas, the defense has been rejected. Thus, in the *Philadelphia National Bank* merger case, the defendants contended that only through merger could certain local Philadelphia banks compete more effectively for large loans with out-of-state banks. The Supreme Court rejected this defense, stating:

> If anticompetitive effects in one market could be justified by procompetitive consequences in another, the logical upshot would be that every firm in an industry could, without violating §7 embark on a series of mergers that would make it in the end as large as the industry leader. For if all the commercial banks in the Philadelphia area merged into one, it would be smaller than the largest bank in New York City. This is not a case, plainly, where two small firms in a market propose to merge in order to be able to compete more successfully with the leading firms in that market.[28]

Consequently, it appears that the countervailing power defense is not likely to be efficacious unless it can be used as a rebuttal to a contention that the merger will be likely to lessen competition in the market. The possibility that this lessening of competition in one market area could lead to an increase in competition in other markets simply has not been accepted.

In the context of a hypothetical merger of two health maintenance organizations, it might be anticipated that if the HMOs could demonstrate that only through their consolidation could they compete effectively with other, larger HMOs, then the consolidation might not be likely to lessen competition in the market area. In this event, the consolidation need not violate any rule of law. If, however, the consolidation would not help stimulate competition through countervailing power in the local market, but might allow the larger, unified HMO to extend its competitive influence into new and more distant markets, then this aspect of countervailing power, although beneficial to the state of competition in other markets, probably would not save the merger from offending Section 7 in the local market immediately affected by that consolidation.

The Failing Company Defense

The basic evil from which conclusions of anticompetitive results are reached in any merger is the removal of a market factor, *i.e.,* the acquired company. However, if that market factor can be shown to have been on the verge of removing itself by simply failing as an enterprise, then the primary reason for the application of anticonsolidation rules of law would seem to be lacking. Where the reason for the rule ceases to exist, the rule also should cease to exist.

This general tenet of rational application of the laws has not gone unnoticed by the courts, and consequently the "failing company defense" has been developed. This in fact is one of the more frequently proffered and more frequently successful defenses when a consolidation is challenged. The burden the consolidating companies must meet to rely successfully upon this theory, however, is not an easy one, in part because the defense requires the demonstration of more than its name might imply.

The failing company defense was first developed by the Supreme Court in a 1930 case involving the merger of two shoe manufacturing companies.[29] In analyzing the merger, the court described the very distressed market situation of one of the companies, concluding that it had reached a point where it no longer could pay its debts as they came due. The company faced insolvency and involuntary liquidation. Its recovery appeared unlikely and it had found no other prospective purchasers. Recognizing all of these factors, the officers, stockholders, and creditors of the company made what the court concluded was a good faith and well-informed decision to sell its stock to a rival shoe manufacturer. The court held that under these circumstances the consolidation did not offend the antitrust laws.

The court's final language in reaching this conclusion seems particularly appropriate:

> In the light of the case thus disclosed of a corporation with resources so depleted and the prospect of rehabilitation so remote that it faced the grave probability of a business failure with resulting loss to its stockholders and injury to the communities where its clients were operat[ing], we hold that the purchase of its capital stock by a competitor (there being no other prospective purchaser), not with a purpose to lessen competition, but to facilitate the accumulated business of the purchaser and with the effect of mitigating seriously injurious consequences otherwise probable, is not in contemplation of law prejudicial to the public and does not substantially lessen competition or restrain commerce within the intent of the Clayton Act.[30]

The failing company defense has been interpreted narrowly by the courts, and the burden on the defendant remains a very strict one of demonstrating that the acquired company is in a serious, even precarious, financial position, suffering an irreversible trend with a grave probability that failure will ensue, and that there is no reasonable, possible, or feasible alternative. The Supreme Court has gone so far as to require that where a purportedly failing company is acquired by a competitor or firm in the same industry, the firms thus united must demonstrate not only the failing nature of the acquired firm, but that the acquiring firm was the only available buyer. If another person or group might be interested in the purchase, then that economic unit might have been preserved and not lost in the consolidation. This rule has been applied in at least one consolidation case involving not only Section 7 of the Clayton Act, but also Sections 1 and 2 of the Sherman Act, where the consolidation resulted in a local monopoly.[31]

Where a local health care provider may be facing an irreversible trend leading inevitably to failure, it may be an insufficient defense to a challenge of the acquisition of the failing entity by another local provider simply to contend that the failing company was likely to disappear from the market place. The company on the verge of failing first must make a good faith, and perhaps exhaustive, effort to find another purchaser or some alternative means of staying alive. Only when these alternatives have been explored and prove unavailing should the failing company anticipate a valid defense to a challenged consolidation with another local provider. In spite of the difficulties in invoking this defense successfully, consolidation does appear to be one viable means of preserving licensed bed capacity in a geographic area encountering individual hospital failures. In this context, the failing company defense is not so much the addition of a caveat from the general standards of the Clayton and Sherman Acts as it is a way of demonstrating that in the long run, competition in the market is not being reduced and only beneficial results are foreseeable.

The Weak Competitor Defense

The failing company defense demonstrates the judicial recognition that statistical representations of a corporation's past activities, including its traditional market share and competitive posture, may not offer a fair description of its present and probable future market position. It also is entirely possible that a company may not be failing or may not otherwise meet the tests required to fulfill the failing company defense, and yet the mere statistical demonstration of its past sales or market share may be misleading.

For example, where a market can be demonstrated to be undergoing major changes in the nature of services or products offered to consumers, or where factors such as long-term contracts operate to preclude a company from actually competing with others while not necessarily impacting upon its statistical market share, or where a company's future prospects are much bleaker than its past and present statistics would indicate, the acquisition of that company might be assumed to have less of an anticompetitive impact than a traditional statistical analysis otherwise would indicate. Again, this type of defense is not so much a departure from the statutory standard of avoiding a substantial lessening of competition as it is a recognition that simplified statistical tests often proffered by the government or other plaintiffs, and almost as often accepted by the courts, sometimes may indicate false anticompetitive impact or may exaggerate the true effect a particular consolidation is likely to have.

Since this type of defense does not depart from statutory standards, it does appear to be entirely valid and has been accepted and even explained in detail by the Supreme Court. In particular, when a company engaged in deep-mining of coal acquired, through stock purchases, the control of a strip-mining company, the Department of Justice challenged the merger as a violation of Section 7 of the Clayton Act.[32] Aside from disputes on the nature of the market, both in terms of geography and in terms of the distinction between deep mining and strip mining, the government's statistical analysis demonstrated that the companies held market shares large enough to create a presumption that the acquisition would lessen competition substantially. Perhaps even more significant, the government demonstrated that the number of coal producing firms in the geographic area had decreased by almost 73 percent during a recent ten-year period. Consequently, there existed the significant trend toward greater concentration in this industry to which the courts historically have been sensitive.

In spite of what might be considered a relatively strong initial showing by the government, both the lower court and the Supreme Court concluded that the acquisition did not violate the antitrust laws. The Supreme Court said the reason for this conclusion was, in part, the consideration of factors unique to the mining industry. The court said the government's statistical showing was not questioned and, under ordinary circumstances, the showing would have supported a finding that the industry was suffering from undue concentration. It added that a merger must be viewed functionally in the context of each particular industry. Statistics reflecting the shares of market control by certain industry leaders, such as the parties in this case, offered one index of market power, it noted. But it said a further examination of the market, including its structure, its history, and its probable future, was required to put the statistics in the proper perspective and to judge the probable anticompetitive effect of the merger.

The court ruled that the structure, history, and probable future of the coal mining industry and the parties demonstrated that the statistics offered a misleading view of the impact of the acquisition. It found that analysis of the industry's history demonstrated that over time the companies in question had become much more dependent upon long-term contracts under which co-producers promised to meet the needs of purchasers, primarily electric utilities, for a fixed period of time and at a predetermined price. The contracts offered the stability both the purchaser and the seller required, and ultimately benefited the consumer. When a particular coal producer entered into such a long-term contract, however, its production statistics might not accurately reflect its position as a competitor in the market. This aberration from statistical analysis, the court said, required consideration of competitive position apart from the overall statistics in order to help determine the probable impact of the acquisition.

The Supreme Court explained the basic rationale for relying so frequently upon statistical analysis of production and market share figures in determining the probable future impact of a particular consolidation. In essence, the court said, the unstated assumption is simply that a company that has maintained a certain share of a market in the past will continue to do so in the immediate future, or at least would have continued to do so but for the acquisition in question. Thus, the court pointed out, it is important to recognize that the statistical analyses are not of value because of what they actually show, *i.e.*, past market position, but rather for what they predict, *i.e.*, competitive posture in the future. Where a company's future then can be demonstrated to be other than what past statistics would indicate, the value of the statistical analysis so often relied upon by the government is lost.

In the mining case, the defendants were able to demonstrate that the acquired company held very few reserves of coal relative to its competitors and to its past production. Consequently, although the company had been a major market factor in the past, the court held that there appeared good reason to believe it would not be such a large factor in the future. The acquired company's size as a producer simply did not properly reflect this weakness in its posture as a competitor. This factor went directly to the question of whether a future lessening of competition was probable, the court ruled, and significantly helped to validate the defendants' contention of the legality of this acquisition.

A particularly good description of the generalized rule that may be applicable in this type of situation was offered by a federal court of appeals in examining the impact of the acquisition of one paper manufacturing corporation by another. Although the acquisition, which was challenged by the Federal Trade Commission, ultimately was determined to be illegal, the court well states the appropriate analysis:

> We now come to the question whether, on the assumptions we have here made, it could be said by the [Federal Trade] Commission that "the effect of such acquisition may be substantially to lessen competition, or to tend to create a monopoly." To answer it we must necessarily consider what the record shows as to the total competitive picture in this relevant area with respect to these products prior to the acquisition. If the acquisition took out of the market a concern whose total sales and competitive impact was so small relative to all sales and all competition in the market that it lacked real importance, then the acquisition can not be said to affect competition in a substantial manner.[33]

Although the court in this case proceeded along a statistical analysis, its statement of the general test was useful. In essence, the analyst must consider both the sales of the concern in question and its competitive impact, which need not coincide with its sales. If this competitive impact is considered in the context of both present and probable future impact of that company on the market, this part of the analysis is complete.

In the context of the health care industry, coal reserves and other such depleting resources are not likely to be a major factor. Long-term requirements contracts, however, could become important, for example, when a hospital has a long-term contract to provide bed services to health maintenance organizations or other entities. Under the same type of theory, if the health maintenance organization had been a major market factor in the past by virtue of contracts to provide services for particular employers and if, for example, some of those employers now proposed to leave the area or to provide for their employees through other means, this general weakness of future prospects for the HMO should constitute a defense to a presumption of anticompetitive impact resulting from its acquisition.

In general, this type of defensive theory should not be overlooked by any provider when analyzing the substantiality of the anticompetitive effect of any consolidation. The health care industry constantly is undergoing changes in its structure and its performance, and the past need not be taken as a reflection of the future, nor can the competitive posture of particular organizations in the industry always be described fairly by a simple statistical analysis.

Defenses Based on the Relevant Market Definition

Whenever a challenge to a proposed or completed consolidation is premised upon the assertion that anticompetitive results will follow from the creation of a company with an unduly large market share, or from the elimination of a company with a market share that made it a significant competitive factor, these assertions in turn must be based on certain definitions of the market to which the shares refer. Any statistical analysis of market shares can be made only after first defining both the appropriate product or service market and the appropriate geographic market.

In virtually all of the cases described in this chapter, the courts have been required to resolve disputes between the parties regarding the definition of the market before attempting to determine the impact of the consolidation upon that market. Frequently, and particularly where it is asserted that the consolidation is of a horizontal nature, the definition of the market may be the key to defending the case and in turn may produce the most hotly contested issues. In general, the plaintiff may be assumed to seek a market definition that demonstrates the most substantial anticompetitive impact resulting from the consolidation. The defendant, predictably, seeks just the opposite.

The Supreme Court has explained that the relevant market in the product or service sense is determined by the reasonable interchangeability of use between the product or service and the purported substitutes for it.[34] It is further possible, the court has said, that within one such market there may exist numerous submarkets, determined by examining such practical conditions as industry or public recognition of a submarket as a separate economic entity, any peculiar characteristics or uses of the service or product, any unique facilities used in providing the service or making the product, the distinctions between customers in the market, and specializations of vendors in the market.

The determination of the geographic market relevant to analysis of a consolidation has been held to be the area in which the competitive effect of the consolidation will be direct and immediate.[35]

In this context, there would appear to be many opportunities to demonstrate the idiosyncrasies of the health care industry. Numerous health care providers may appear at first to be in the same general market. When specialties, areas of emphasis, specialized patient and physician populations, and other factors are considered, however, submarkets and market definition matters may be expected to be important factors in the analysis of virtually any consolidation in this industry.

Government Regulation As A Defense

Certain aspects of government regulation can lead to absolute defenses from the application of the antitrust laws. As previously explained, where the state, as part of a valid state program, compels certain conduct, the antitrust laws may not be applied to that conduct, by virtue of the state action defense. Where the application of the antitrust laws is repugnant to the operation of another federal regulatory scheme, those laws may be deemed inapplicable under the doctrine of implied repeal. Similarly, where conduct that otherwise would be scrutinized under the antitrust laws must be evaluated first by an administrative agency under a valid regulatory program, the doctrine of primary jurisdiction may usurp that first level of scrutiny from the courts.

Instances in which governmental regulation of the health care industry may replace the application of the antitrust laws entirely are considered later in this work. It is possible, however, that even where the governmental regulatory scheme does not entirely usurp the application of the antitrust laws, the impact of that regulatory program may make certain traditional antitrust doctrines and principles inapplicable. This is particularly true insofar as prosecutors may attempt to apply traditional antitrust doctrines, such as the potential competition doctrine, to health care consolidations.

An example of the effect of a governmental regulatory scheme on the application of traditional antitrust principles in a merger situation was explained by the Supreme Court in a case involving the merger of two banks in the State of Washington.[36] Although the health care industry, of course, was not involved in this case, the regulatory scheme and its impact on antitrust principles appears to be directly analogous to foreseeable events in the health care industry.

In the bank merger situation, the court analyzed the merger along traditional lines, determining the relevant geographic and product or service markets and considering the size and market position of each bank. Each operated in various parts of the state, but the merger would give the acquiring company offices in areas in which it previously had not operated. The prosecution contended, and the court agreed, that the potential competition doctrine was appropriate in determining whether the merger had an anticompetitive impact by removing the acquiring company as a potential competitor. In essence, the acquiring company might have extended its operations into those other parts of the state but, after the acquisition, it would not have the incentive to do so because it simply was acquiring active businesses in the new territories.

Upon further analysis, however, when the court attempted to apply the traditional potential competition doctrine to the commercial banking market in the State of Washington, it found the doctrine inapplicable because commercial banks in the state were required to obtain governmental approval before opening offices in new territories. Consequently, the court held it was unrealistic to suggest that the acquiring bank simply might open branch offices independently in new market areas because the openings would require this governmental approval first. Thus, taking into account the extensive regulation of the banking industry, the court concluded that the potential competition doctrine did not indicate the likelihood that the spirit of competition in the market would be lessened substantially by the merger.

The rule in this case appears to be directly analogous to situations that might be encountered in the health care industry. Certificate of need requirements make a virtual mockery of the potential competition doctrine in the industry. This is particularly true in an era during which excess capacity so often is blamed for perceived excessive health care costs that any new entry that could be characterized as competitive to virtually anything already existing is relatively unlikely to receive a certificate of need. Consequently, if a proposed merger does offer particular economies or other benefits to the patient population, it would seem unreasonable to apply a traditional potential competition analysis, depriving the consumers of the benefits of the merger merely in the interest of preserving illusory potential competition.

PREMERGER NOTIFICATION REQUIREMENTS

Section 7a of the Clayton Act[37] provides that persons intending to engage in acquisitions that meet certain criteria must first file notice of that intention with both the Federal Trade Commission and the Department of Justice, and must then wait for a stated period, generally 30 days. This gives the FTC and Justice the opportunity to seek to stop the acquisition before it is consummated.

The basic criteria for determining whether the proposed acquisition is subject to the premerger notification rules are:

1. If either the acquiring party or the acquired party is engaged in commerce or in an activity affecting commerce (thus going beyond the ''in commerce'' only application of Section 7 of the Clayton Act), and
2. If the acquired party is engaged in manufacturing and has net sales or total assets of at least $10 million and the acquiring party has total assets or net sales of at least $100 million, or
3. If the acquired party is not engaged in manufacturing but has total assets of at least $10 million and the acquiring party has total assets or net sales of at least $100 million, or
4. The acquired party has net sales or total assets of at least $100 million and the acquiring party has total assets or net sales of at least $10 million, and
5. The acquisition will cause the acquiring party to hold either 15 percent or more of the lease securities or assets of the acquired party or to hold total lease securities and assets of the acquired party in excess of $15 million.

The statute provides certain exemptions from the notification requirements. The exemptions most likely to apply to the health care industry, either now or in the future, include those for transactions specifically exempted from the antitrust laws by federal statute if approved by a federal agency (although the agency still is required to make informational filings with the FTC and the Department of Justice). Other exemptions relate to transactions in the ordinary course of business and acquisitions solely for investment.

The FTC has published detailed rules on providing notification where required, including forms for use in filing.[38]

NOTES

1. *See, Modern Health Care,* August 1978, at 8.

2. *See, Modern Health Care,* April 1978, at 46.

3. *See, Hospitals,* Feb. 16, 1973 at 60; *Harron v. United Hospital Center, Inc.,* 522 F.2d 1133 (4th Cir. 1975).

4. *See, e.g., Hospitals,* Jan. 1, 1979, at 82.

5. *See, Forum,* September 1978, at 19.

6. 15 U.S.C. § 18.

7. 15 U.S.C. § 44; the definition of corporations subject to FTC jurisdiction specifically excludes those not organized for their own profit or the profit of the members; but see, *Philadelphia Nat'l Bank,* 374 U.S. 321.

8. This seemingly curious dichotomy was created by the 1950 amendment to § 7, which for the first time inserted language restricting acquisition of assets. Prior to this amendment, the statute applied only to consolidations achieved through purchases of stock. The amendment, however, also added the requirement that, in the case of an asset acquisition, the acquiring corporation would be subject to FTC jurisdiction.

9. 422 U.S. 271, 95 S.Ct. 2150 (1975); efforts were underway, however, to change the applicable standards to "affecting commerce."

10. 95 S.Ct. 2155-2156 (1975).

11. 189 F. Supp. 153 (D.C.N.Y. 1960).

12. 189 F. Supp. 181-182.

13. *FTC v. Lancaster Colony Corp., Inc.,* 434 F. Supp. 1088 (S.D.N.Y. 1977).

14. *See, e.g., U.S. v. Philadelphia Nat'l Bank,* 374 U.S. 321, 83 S.Ct. 1715 (1963).

15. *U.S. v. First Nat'l Bank and Trust Company of Lexington,* 376 U.S. 665, 84 S.Ct. 1033 (1964).

16. *American Medicorp, Inc. v. Humana, Inc.,* 445 F. Supp. 589 (E.D.Pa. 1977).

17. 562 F.2d 280 (4th Cir. 1977), *vacated,* 98 S.Ct. 1642.

18. *Hospitals,* "Medical Staffs Merge," February 16, 1973, at 60 (*supra,* note 3).

19. *Supra,* note 15.

20. *U.S. v. Von's Grocery Co.,* 384 U.S. 270, 86 S.Ct. 1478 (1966).

21. *U.S. v. Pabst Brewing Co.,* 384 U.S. 546, 86 S.Ct. 1665 (1966).

22. *Supra,* note 15.

23. *See Supra,* note 5, at 20.

24. 329 F.Supp. 919 (E.D.Pa. 1971).

25. *See especially,* the appendix to the concurring opinion of Justice Douglas in *U.S. v. Pabst Brewing Co., supra,* note 21 at 1669, wherein he relates Art Buchwald's description of the ultimate corporate consolidation.

26. F.T.C. v. Proctor & Gamble Co., 386 U.S. 568,580; 87 S.Ct. 1224 (1967).

27. *See* discussion of arguments in favor of economies as a defense in vertical merger cases in Sullivan, *Antitrust,* at 667-669 (West, 1977).

28. *Supra,* note 14, at 1745.

29. *International Shoe Co. v. FTC,* 280 U.S. 291, 50 S.Ct. 89 (1930).

30. *Supra,* note 29, at 302-303.

31. *Citizen Publishing Co. v. U.S.,* 394 U.S. 131, 89 S.Ct. 927 (1969).

32. *U.S. v. General Dynamics Corp.,* 415 U.S. 486, 94 S.Ct. 1186 (1974).

33. *Crown Zellerbach Corp. v. FTC,* 296 F.2d 800 (9th Cir. 1961).

34. *Brown Shoe Co., v. U.S.,* 370 U.S. 294, 82 S.Ct. 1502 (1962).

35. *U.S. v. Marine Bancorporation,* 418 U.S. 602, 94 S.Ct. 2856 (1974).

36. *Supra,* note 34.

37. 15 U.S.C. §18a.

38. Federal Register, July 31, 1978, 43 C.F.R. 33451.

Chapter 5

The Role of
Trade Associations

Because of their common concerns and interests, persons engaged in similar or competitive business activities have joined in cooperative groups to seek solutions to their problems, at least since medieval craftsmen formed guilds. However, any cooperative venture of competitors may tend to diminish the competition among them, as solutions to problems and other operational decisions may be the product of consultation and agreement rather than individual analysis and judgment. Since the antitrust laws express the general view that individual decision making ordinarily is desirable and that pluralism is at the heart of our economy and basic to its efficiency, the propriety of associations of competitors has been questionable at times. While today no one seriously disputes that trade associations play legitimate roles, it is just as clear that some associational activities are forbidden and that, even when the functions are proper, the association must be cautious that it does not pursue forbidden paths toward given ends, whether or not those objectives themselves are forbidden.

Trade associations have many legitimate functions in the health care field. There are horizontally related entities such as the American Hospital Association and professional societies such as the American Medical Association. Shared service organizations—entities with similar needs that unite to perform joint functions such as group purchasing—can take various forms, including that of an association.

Trade associations and professional societies engage in many of the same activities, including collecting and disseminating information, representing the interests of their memberships to the government and to the public, standardizing and certifying the quality of the goods or services provided, establishing codes of ethical conduct for their members, and advertising for the members or enhancing their public image. The purposes of shared service organizations generally are limited to providing their members with specific economic advantages, such as cheaper materials or goods through cooperative buying.

There are two basic ways in which trade association activities may violate the antitrust laws. First, the association may engage in activities that themselves are unlawful, such as price fixing, allocating markets, or otherwise restraining trade unreasonably. Second, even if an association provides a lawful benefit to its members, it may violate the law by discriminating against nonmember competitors in the course of helping its members. In this chapter, both "unlawful conduct" and "exclusionary" anticompetitive practices are discussed.

As with so many aspects of applying the antitrust laws to health care, a consideration that often has arisen in challenging association activities is whether the disputed conduct created the requisite impact on interstate commerce. As noted previously, the defense that challenged conduct is not subject to scrutiny under the federal antitrust laws because of a lack of impact on interstate commerce is becoming less viable as courts and litigants find new ways to demonstrate the interrelationships between local conduct and interstate commerce. Such interrelationships often are particularly demonstrable in the context of association activities.

Many trade and professional associations are interstate in nature and thus may perform functions directly within the flow of interstate commerce. Even local associations may engage in interstate purchases and thus be "in commerce," as well as "affecting commerce" through local activities that have interstate repercussions. In a 1977 trade association antitrust case, for example, a group of individuals charged that the National Board for Respiratory Therapy and others engaged in testing and certification programs had helped cause hospitals to refuse to hire uncertified therapists.[1] The defendants contended that the conduct did not affect interstate commerce sufficiently to allow the application of the Sherman Act. The court concluded, however, that the following aspects of the conduct were sufficient to allow the case to proceed under federal jurisdiction:

1. The defendants advertised on a multistate basis.
2. The defendants administered examinations on a multistate basis.
3. The certification and registration requirements caused an increase in prices.

Other typical aspects of association conduct are equally capable of impacting upon interstate commerce, or even being a part of interstate commerce. The liberalizing of these jurisdictional requirements thus is of substantial significance to all who participate in trade and professional associations.

RESTRICTIONS ON ASSOCIATIONS' BENEFITS

Trade associations frequently have restricted memberships and criteria for determining membership eligibility. Presumably, membership is perceived to benefit their members, since otherwise there would be no reason for associating.

However, when an association adopts a restrictive membership policy or otherwise limits important benefits to members only, it may violate the prohibition against restraints of trade in Section 1 of the Sherman Act.

Reasonable Membership Constraints

While the safest practice for a trade association is to open its membership to all competitors and even potential competitors in the industry,[2] an association may establish requirements that are reasonable in light of its purpose and functions, assuming that the purpose of the restrictions is not anticompetitive. An example of an anticompetitive restriction might be denying entry on the basis of membership in a competing association.[3] The standard applied is the "rule of reason,"[4] and courts consider a variety of factors relevant to whether a membership requirement is reasonable or arbitrary.

The degree to which a trade or professional association is required not to discriminate against competitors depends generally upon the importance of membership in the group. For example, if membership or some benefit it confers, such as certification, is required for one to be active in a trade, business, or profession, then the association's standards and procedures for granting that favored status must meet a higher test of equitability than if membership has no competitive importance.[5] When membership is particularly important, even a group of essentially joint venturers may be required to open its rolls.[6] If, for instance, participation in a shared service organization were practically necessary in order to function in a market, then membership in the organization would need to be open to actual or potential competitors, unless other circumstances made restrictions necessary or at least reasonable.

Freedom of association, in itself, is a constitutionally protected right.[7] Persons ordinarily are permitted to associate with whomever they desire. Membership in a trade association, however, goes beyond basic constitutional rights, and therefore such groups are allowed to establish reasonable criteria. At the heart of most membership issues is the question of what requirements are "reasonable" in a particular context, since even if membership or other privileges are required to compete, the group may deny the privileges if the process for determining when to deny membership is reasonable and if the association makes its decisions on the basis of reasonable standards rather than to restrain trade.[8] For example, granting certification or membership privileges on the basis of skill is valid if the required level of ability and the testing procedures are reasonable.[9]

Physicians, Nonphysicians, and Specialists

Local medical societies sometimes have adopted rules and regulations that discriminate against health care professionals who have not attended schools certified by the American Medical Association or who have not graduated with the degree of Medical Doctor (as differentiated from the degree of Doctor of Osteopathy) and prevent them from obtaining all of the benefits that accrue to the profession they have chosen. Associations of dentists, chiropractors, and psychologists have adopted similar rules and regulations. When the societies create barriers to entry for those who otherwise are qualified to engage in a particular occupation, antitrust questions are raised.

The types of questions that must be considered are the reasons for such rules:

- Has there been a joining together purposely to exclude a particular segment of health care professionals?
- Has the action been taken to prevent those individuals from successfully practicing their professions?
- Is membership in the local, state, or national society an economic necessity so that without membership the nonmembers cannot compete effectively for business with members?

If the answer to any of these questions is in the affirmative, then the circumstances will be subject to close antitrust scrutiny.

The probable effect of being denied membership in a county society is that a large portion of the expected practice of a physician cannot be maintained because of the concurrent denial of staff privileges in certain hospitals,[10] and some individuals denied membership in societies vital to the successful practice of their profession have brought legal actions against the groups and their officers. Several cases have been instituted by persons excluded from membership in specialized trade associations in the health care industry, and some of these cases have included allegations of antitrust violations.[11] Most such cases seek court orders to the effect that the plaintiff is entitled to membership and the benefits afforded members of the societies that had sought to exclude that individual. Damages resulting from unreasonable exclusions also may be available.

Nonphysician professional associations in the health care industry also have been defendants in antitrust suits based on membership requirements. Plaintiff dentists, in a 1977 case in Arizona, alleged that local and state dental associations required membership in the American Dental Association as a prerequisite to membership in either the local or state association.[12] The questions actually addressed by the court, however, concerned whether the alleged restraint of trade affected interstate commerce and whether dentistry was a "learned profession" and thus exempt from the Sherman Act.[13] To practice dentistry in the state, in this instance, membership was not required in either the state or local association. However, members were entitled to participate in continuing education programs, group insurance, referral plans, and exchanges of information with other dentists. The plaintiffs claimed that unless they joined the American Dental Association, they would be prevented from participating in activities or enjoying the benefits of the local and state associations, which they wanted to join without the required national association membership.

The court found the requisite interstate commerce present because the programs, coordination, and membership of the American Dental Association were multistate in origin. Funds crossed from local societies to the national one and from the national society to others. In addition, by adopting the reasoning of the discussion of the "learned profession" exemption in the Supreme Court opinions in *Goldfarb v. Virginia State Bar*[14] and *Cantor v. Detroit Edison Co.*, [15] the court found that "neither an expansive 'learned profession' nor equally expansive 'state action' exemption exists," but the court did explain that dentistry was not merely a commercial enterprise.

On the defendant association's motion to dismiss the action, the court explained that for a rule or regulation to survive a Sherman Act challenge, it must be of some benefit to the public. In this instance, it said, the challenged regulation relating to membership in the American Dental Association was not designed to improve dental services to the public. Therefore, the court allowed the plaintiff to go forward with the lawsuit.

CERTIFICATION AND ACCREDITATION

The power to accredit and certify is particularly important for the professions, including the health care professions, and associations that accredit institutions or certify the capabilities of individuals must do so on the basis of reasonable and relevant standards.[16] Certification commonly is an adjunct of membership, and because of the importance of membership in a professional society or an accrediting association, courts have made clear their jurisdiction to consider the validity of entry procedures under the antitrust and other laws, even while approving the standards and procedures of the associations and societies.[17]

An association, particularly one with regulatory or quasi-regulatory power, also may deny certification unreasonably when it expands its domain of control beyond activities that are legitimately within its sphere of influence. For example, while practicing law without a license from a state bar may be illegal, the state bar may have broad ideas about what constitutes the practice of law. The same may be true with regard to the practice of medicine.

If the licensing of the occupation is the function of a state agency, the issues may not involve the antitrust laws directly since the conduct may be insulated as state action,[18] but the antitrust laws clearly would be applicable to a private association forbidding or restraining economic conduct of persons outside the normal scope of the organization's activities.[19]

Certification in the Medical Industry

Those engaged in specialties and subspecialties in health care have formed separate associations that serve a variety of functions for their memberships. Some associations offer advanced training or continuing education, others provide opportunities to socialize with individuals in the same profession. Associations also certify for practice individuals deemed qualified to engage in a particular type of work. When only one organization exists for a profession, and that association is responsible for certifying the qualification of individuals for practice, the group has effective monopoly power over that profession. An individual denied membership in an association that certifies the qualifications of individuals seeking to become members is effectively prevented from obtaining employment in that chosen profession.

Numerous courts have considered the various reasons why individuals are not accepted for membership in associations and have dealt with the constitutional issues raised by rejections.[20] The more difficult cases are those in which the certifying board must rate the qualifications of the individuals. Courts have been called upon to determine whether the association criteria are consistent with the antitrust laws and whether they encourage or discourage competition in the profession.[21]

Some specialties require that applicants for certification pass an examination. In a case concerning the certification of respiratory therapists, the plaintiffs failed the required examination.[22] They sued the associations responsible for certification and a hospital that refused to hire respiratory therapists unless they were registered or certified. The antitrust claim was based upon the defendants' refusal to deal[23] by declining to employ individuals unless they passed the examination. The plaintiffs also charged that the association monopolized[24] the pool of available therapists so the hospitals would hire only those certified and registered by the association.

In *Bogus v. American Speech and Hearing Association*,[25] the plaintiffs challenged the association's rule that required the maintenance of membership as a prerequisite to receiving a Certificate of Clinical Competence (CCC). The certificate was issued only by the trade association and was a generally recognized symbol of competence in that profession. In fact, the CCC was considered to be a professional necessity in some employment submarkets for speech pathologists and audiologists. The association would issue the CCC only to those who had completed certain educational and training requirements *and* were dues-paying members of the association. The plaintiff, a speech pathologist who chose not to pay dues to the association after receiving a CCC (and therefore lost the certificate), contended that the association had tied association membership to the issuance of the CCC, in violation of the Sherman Act.

A Federal appellate court essentially validated the plaintiff's theory by permitting the case to go forward to trial rather than dismissing it on procedural grounds. The court ruled:

> A direct purchaser who demonstrates a legitimate economic or business interest in purchasing a desirable or unique tying product or service and who is thereby compelled to purchase as well a tied product or service has standing to challenge the legality of the tie-in. On this record there is sufficient material evidence that plaintiff had a legitimate professional interest in acquiring a CCC at the time she applied for it and first joined ASHA.[26]

The court added that, although the plaintiff's theory was valid, victory at trial would require that she demonstrate: (1) that the association actually conditioned the issuance of the CCC upon maintaining a dues-paying membership in the association; (2) that the amount of commerce affected by the restriction was not insubstantial; and (3) that the CCC was such a sufficiently desirable and unique item that she reasonably believed she was professionally compelled to maintain her association membership.

An additional aspect of association conduct raised occasionally in certification cases is educational requirements. A professional association, for example, may require completion of a certain level of education for certification or for admission to membership. The issue that must be addressed in such cases is the economic importance of the association and whether it is in a monopolistic position. Unless some economic necessity for membership in the association is shown, courts have been unwilling to make a finding of monopolization through educational requirements or any other antitrust violation. Unless membership in the association, or certification by the group, is a requirement for practicing in the profession, courts have been reluctant to give significant deference to a challenger's position.[27]

Certification issues apply not only to individuals but also to entire groups, such as those who attend a particular school. Consequently, lawsuits may be pursued by representatives of such groups. A private dental school, for example, brought an antitrust suit against an association of orthodontists, an association of dentists, and certain individuals.[28] The school did not claim to certify its students as qualified orthodontists, but it did claim to teach specialty techniques to practicing dentists so they could expand their general dentistry practices. The plaintiff, the United States Dental Institute (USDI), contended that the defendants had effectuated a boycott of the school in order to enable the associations and their members to monopolize the practice of orthodontia through the following steps·

> (1) defendants acted to prevent USDI from receiving approval from the State of Illinois to operate as a post-secondary educational facility; when such certification was awarded to USDI, defendants sought to have the Illinois Superintendent of Public Instruction revoke such approval; (2) defendants refused to publish USDI advertisements seeking qualified faculty, as well as listings of USDI courses in the Journal of the ADA; (3) defendants issued certain "Guidelines for Continuing Dental Education" which sought to eliminate USDI and any other for-profit group as a source of continuing dental education, by withholding ADA accreditation; (4) defendants issued advisory ethics opinions in which they declared it to be unethical for a dentist to sponsor, conduct or participate as a teacher in a non-ADA approved program, for the purpose of discouraging potential faculty members; (5) defendants adopted restrictive standards on general practitioner dentists effectively preventing them from performing orthodontia services, while at the same time restricting their opportunities for further training in orthodontia techniques.[29]

The court held that the cause of action was adequate to allow the plaintiff to go forward and prove its case at trial because: (1) the contentions demonstrated the requisite impact on interstate commerce; (2) there was no learned profession exemption to protect the conduct; (3) the contentions demonstrated that the defendants were not motivated solely by a sense of duty to protect professionals and the public from substandard practices; (4) the conduct in issue would protect a monopolistic position and enable the defendants to charge higher rates for their services; and (5) the immunity for efforts to influence legislative action would not protect conduct intended to interfere directly with the plaintiff's business.

Associations of individual medical professionals present only one general form of group that may lead to antitrust violations in the health care industry. While associations may restrict membership, prevent certification, and thereby prevent individuals from engaging in their chosen professions, hospitals themselves may act as associations and, through their denial of rights to staff privilege or in other ways, individuals may not be entitled to practice, and hospitals may be subject to antitrust violations. The antitrust implications pertain both to individuals and hospitals. The most common situation arises when a hospital prevents a physician from obtaining staff privileges. Association conduct becomes a concurrent concern when a hospital's refusal to grant such a privilege is based on pressure from a county medical society or other organized trade or professional associations.[30]

Association Boycotts of Nonmedical Doctors

Medical associations have been accused of directing anticompetitive efforts at nonmembers or at groups that may compete for patients but that are licensed for different specialties. For example, a professional society might try to prevent chiropractors or podiatrists from competing with the work of a physician.

The most litigated subject in this area has concerned the failure to allow graduates of colleges of osteopathy, later certified as medical doctors, to become members of medical societies or of medical staffs of hospitals. The seminal case concerning osteopaths and alleged boycotts by a medical society is *Falcone v. Middlesex County Medical Society*.[31] In that 1961 New Jersey case, the plaintiff, a Dr. Falcone, had received a full medical course and had been graduated with the degree of Doctor of Osteopathy. He passed the medical examination prescribed by the New Jersey State Board of Medical Examiners and was licensed to practice medicine and surgery in the state. The school Dr. Falcone had attended originally, the Philadelphia College of Osteopathy, was not approved as a medical college by the American Medical Association. He later received an M.D. degree from the College of Medicine at the University of Milan, a medical college approved by the AMA.

The Middlesex County Medical Society, however, refused to admit Dr. Falcone as an active member, notwithstanding the fact that it had no written policy precluding membership of a physician who had been graduated from an AMA-approved medical school, regardless of the degree held at the time of original licensure. Rather, the society applied an unwritten rule requiring that members attend a four-year course of study at an AMA-approved school, and Dr. Falcone had failed to meet only that unwritten standard. The society's denial of membership resulted in Dr. Falcone's being terminated from the medical staff of the Middlesex General Hospital and St. Peter's General Hospital, both of which required society membership as a requisite to medical staff privileges. The court, in fact, termed the control the local society had over the practice of medicine in the area a "virtual monopoly." Dr. Falcone sought the assistance of the state medical society, but it refused to intervene on his behalf. The American Medical Association took a similar position, stating that it lacked jurisdiction.

In reaching its decision compelling the society to admit Dr. Falcone to membership, the court ruled the county medical society to be an association that affected the public by its activities and about which the public knew and cared. The court discussed the proper role for the society and stated:

> Public policy strongly dictates that this power should not be unbridled but should be viewed judicially as a fiduciary power to be exercised in reasonable and lawful manner for the advancement of the interests of

the medical profession and the public generally; the evidence firmly
displays that here it was not so exercised . . .[32]

Here, the court found that the monopoly power of the county society was an
overwhelming factor in placing an individual in a position to practice medicine
in a certain locale and that society membership was an actual "economic necessity" for a practicing physician.

The link between a hospital and a county medical society, as well as an alternative approach to avoiding the anticompetitive effects of restrictive society
membership requirements, was illuminated further in another New Jersey case,
in 1963, involving an osteopath's application for membership on the courtesy
medical staff of a private hospital.[33] In this instance, an individual who had been
graduated from a college of osteopathy was given an unqualified license to practice medicine and surgery in several states. He also was the only physician in a
particular area in the state and served as the physician for various companies and
schools. The plaintiff applied for courtesy staff privileges in the local hospital—
the only one in the metropolitan area. The request was denied because a provision in the hospital bylaws stated that all courtesy staff members must be graduates of a medical school approved by the American Medical Association and
also must be members of the county medical society, the requisite society membership being unavailable to osteopaths.

Contrary to the approach taken by Dr. Falcone in the earlier case, the plaintiff
here sued to compel the hospital to disregard its bylaws and grant the requested
staff privileges, rather than suing the medical society to compel admission. The
court's approach to this alternative type of request was almost identical to, and
in fact relied upon, the analysis in *Falcone,* and reached a similar result. Although the hospital contended that its private nature exempted it from scrutiny
over its own rules of admission to staff privileges, the court declared that where
a hospital enjoyed a substantially monopolistic position in an area, it was in no
position to claim immunity from public supervision and control. Consequently,
the court ruled, the same type of reasoning that permits courts to compel trade
associations to grant membership privileges in certain circumstances also permits
those courts to bypass the association and compel the desired incident of membership (here, medical staff privileges).

Much of the reasoning in these cases involved the monopoly position of the
hospital in the community. If the hospital did not have a monopoly, the courts
might not have been as sympathetic to the plaintiffs' arguments. The antitrust
laws protect those harmed economically by an effort to restrain trade. In a community where one institution can restrain the ability of an individual to practice
a chosen profession, that individual would have a better claim, at least under
traditional analysis, than one denied staff privileges in a hospital on the basis of

a county medical society policy and concurrently granted staff privileges in another hospital that chose to ignore the policy. In more recent cases in which all hospitals abide by the dictates of a society, the monopoly argument remains just as viable as in the one-hospital community.

Some cases have been unsuccessful, where, for example, osteopaths were denied membership in a county medical society because of a requirement that all members have completed a four-year course in a medical college[34] (as in *Falcone*), but the plaintiffs failed to demonstrate that the society enjoyed monopoly power or that membership was an economic necessity. Consequently, where membership denials do not interfere materially with the profession of excluded persons, associations continue to enjoy traditionally greater latitude in setting admission and other standards. The courts thus continue to require a showing of economic harm and, if a medical society refuses membership and the effect does not create economic hardship, they are not likely to intervene.[35] Fewer cases are brought now by osteopaths since states have begun according degrees from osteopathic colleges the same status as those leading to an M.D. Osteopaths now are treated as M.D.s and such suits are less likely to arise. Nevertheless, these earlier judicial opinions still are significant because they remain the most frequently followed precedents for group boycotts by trade associations or professional societies in the health care industry.

Other nonphysicians have been confronted with similar boycotts by medical societies. In one instance, a chiropractic institution brought an antitrust action against a city and county medical society and others,[36] charging that the defendants had combined and conspired to prevent the institution from being licensed by the state, which prevented its operation. The plaintiff also contended that the method by which the state licensed medical professionals excluded the practice of chiropractic. Basically, the issue was that the society had monopolized the practice of healing arts.

Since the case was heard back in 1952, the court was concerned primarily with the interstate commerce requirement,[37] and concluded that the only purpose of the alleged monopoly was to limit the practice of chiropractic in that state. The court found the practice to be exclusively local and did not accept the plaintiff's argument that the society had a direct effect upon interstate commerce. Therefore, it held that the effect on such commerce was not enough to bring it within the scope of the Sherman Act. Naturally, because of changes in case law since then, a similar action now could be expected to proceed beyond the jurisdictional issue.

In another antitrust action, chiropractors alleged that a state medical society and a health insurance corporation had conspired to deny health insurance coverage for chiropractic services,[38] which made chiropractic services unattractive to patients. The plaintiffs charged that the defendants had sought to eliminate potential competition from chiropractors. Unlike the earlier case, the plaintiffs here were permitted to proceed rather than being dismissed for procedural reasons.

A 1978 case involving chiropractors was brought under the New Jersey state antitrust statute by a chiropractic society, individual chiropractors, and three individuals who were consumers of chiropractic services.[39] The defendants included a local medical society, the American Medical Association, and hospitals and professional corporations. The plaintiffs accused the defendants of combining to monopolize trade and commerce for the treatment of conditions that both chiropractors and medical doctors could treat. The court, deciding first the question of standing under the state antitrust act,[40] dismissed the claim of the chiropractic society because it was not engaged in business and therefore lacked standing to assert an antitrust claim for money damages under the state act. The plaintiffs claimed they had been forced to go to a doctor of medicine to have x-rays taken because of the alleged conspiracy to monopolize trade in this aspect of health care. The court found that the consumers had suffered injury because the defendants had prohibited them from using chiropractors and instead had required them to use the services of medical doctors, presumably at higher prices.

Although the New Jersey court in that case said it was applying rules equally applicable to federal Sherman Act cases in determining that the chiropractic association lacked standing to bring an antitrust action on behalf of its members, and although another New Jersey court reached the same conclusion in an action on behalf of an optometric association, this is not necessarily the general rule. A federal trial court in 1974, in *Alabama Optometric Association v. Alabama State Board of Health*,[41] explained the more commonly applied rule, to the effect that associations have standing to sue whenever they or their members are injured. The association then may be allowed to pursue an action for the interests of its present members, the interests of the profession generally, and in the interest of those who someday will be members of the profession. It still is possible, however, that distinctions will be made between actions for injunctive relief (such as an order prohibiting defendants from boycotting members of a plaintiff association) and actions for money damages

A somewhat unusual twist involving potential plaintiffs and persons damaged by denial of association memberships is illustrated by the Federal appellate decision in *Elizabeth Hospital v. Richardson*.[42] While this case is rather typical in that it involves the refusal of a local medical society to grant membership to a particular local physician, it is unusual in that the plaintiff was a hospital at which the excluded physician served as chief of staff. The denial of association membership did not result in any denial of hospital staff privileges to the physician, but the hospital charged that the association's refusal to admit its chief of staff caused a loss of patient referrals, which reduced the hospital's patient census correspondingly. Although this case occurred in 1959, before the develop-

ment of modern theories that revised the degree of contacts necessary to constitute interstate commerce, and therefore was dismissed for lack of federal jurisdiction, it does illustrate the extent to which the repercussions of association
conduct may be felt, and the breadth of potential plaintiffs.

DISCIPLINE AND EXPULSION

Related to membership requirements issues are those concerning discipline by
denial of benefits or by expulsion. The legal standards are much the same: associations may expel members or deny benefits for cause if the cause is reasonable and if the relevant procedures also are reasonable. While the grounds for
exclusion thus must not be anticompetitive, if they are in fact reasonable, and if
the procedures also are reasonable, disciplinary exclusion will be lawful even if
it has anticompetitive effects.[43]

Typically, an association invokes its disciplinary process to enforce a code of
ethics or other rules. Assuming that the code or the rules are reasonable,[44] as
with membership, the procedural standards required by law vary directly according to the harm of exclusion or, in other words, with the economic power of the
association. At a minimum, the party facing discipline must be informed of the
charges,[45] but the procedural burden increases if the effect of discipline is severe.
Thus, for example, where an indefinite suspension of a professional golfer from
an association of professional golfers prevented her from pursuing her profession, a court held in 1973 that the decision to suspend her could not be made by
her competitors.[46]

Similar cases have been brought in the health care industry. In one, a dentist
asked a court to declare certain provisions of the local dental society's code of
ethics invalid.[47] The court held that the state law permitted every licensed dentist
to belong to the society. Loss of that membership would deprive the plaintiff of
substantial rights and result in adverse economic consequences.[48] The court declared that the challenged ethical code provisions were invalid and enjoined the
defendant society from taking any action against the plaintiff for violating the
code.

In another action, a medical technologist sought to compel the American Society of Clinical Pathologists to recertify her as a medical technologist.[49] The
plaintiff had violated the society's code of ethics when she accepted a position
in a laboratory not supervised by a medical doctor. The court ruled that judicial
intervention was more likely in the case of individuals seeking reinstatement
following wrongful expulsion rather than simply seeking admission to a society.[50] The court found that certification by the society granted her recognition
and status, and that her loss of certification impaired her standing in the profes-

sion. The court said the society's code deprived the public of obtaining the highest quality of service in laboratories and conflicted with state law and, consequently, no valid basis existed upon which plaintiff could be denied recertification.

ASSOCIATIONS AND BOYCOTTS

While the general rules on joint refusals to deal (group boycotts), were discussed in greater detail in Chapter 1, it should be recalled that an agreement among a group of competitors to refuse to deal with another competitor generally is a *per se* violation of the Sherman Act. Other forms of refusals to deal may not be *per se* offenses, but virtually all are at least suspect until a reasonable basis for the refusal is shown. Since trade and professional associations vigorously advocate the economic interests of their members, they frequently find themselves opposing the interests of competitors or potential competitors. An association, however, should not become a vehicle for a boycott of businesses that are actual or potential competitors of its members.

For example, an association of retailers was prohibited from circulating among its members a list of wholesalers who had sold directly to consumers; even in the absence of an explicit agreement to boycott the listed wholesalers, circulation of such a list implies blacklisting.[51] Such conduct ordinarily is not defensible on the ground that it serves to prevent anticompetitive conduct or other evils and thus is reasonable. The Supreme Court on at least one occasion has taken the view that a private association may not act as a governmental regulatory agency, policing what its members believe to be, or believe should be, violations of the law.[52] Where an association actually is charged by law with a duty to engage in professional regulation or supervision, however, a different analysis may apply.

Boycotts and Barriers to Entry of Prepaid Health Plans

Most of the cases discussed above concern health care professionals faced with barriers to their entry into practice or prohibitions on their engaging in certain types of work. Another cause that has inspired action by medical societies concerns prepaid health plans and other types of relatively innovative ways of providing health care services. Nonfee-for-service health systems, as well as those that emphasize paraprofessional as opposed to physician services, can change the complexion of the health care industry radically. HMOs, without intending to restrict the analysis to plans that are federally qualified as such, are confronted with challenges to their existence by segments of the medical industry. Arguments against HMOs usually assert that they do not encourage physicians to care properly for patients, but instead inspire them to be more cost efficient since the amount patients pay does not grow as the treatment increases.

The control over health services so often enjoyed by the traditional fee-for-service segment of the industry thus might put its members in a position to inhibit the growth of alternative systems through denials of medical society memberships to participant physicians, denials of staff privileges to physicians who attempt to divide their services between the fee-for-service and alternative areas, refusals of admissions to patients under the care of HMO physicians, and even unfavorable reimbursement policies through fee-for-service institutions dominated by Blue Cross and Blue Shield. Where a group of similarly situated professionals, such as fee-for-service physicians, is feared likely to desire to inhibit the development of competitive entities, such as HMOs, then the use of influential trade associations becomes the most likely focus for the fears of the potential (and actual) competitors. Not surprisingly, therefore, actions and investigations of efforts in the fee-for-service segment to inhibit HMO growth have focused on the use of trade associations to achieve such a goal.

In *American Medical Association v. United States,*[53] the first major physician antitrust case addressed by the Supreme Court (1943), the court affirmed the convictions of the AMA and the Medical Society of the District of Columbia for violation of Section 3 of the Sherman Act through a conspiracy to obstruct the operation of a nonprofit corporation that government employees had organized as a prepaid medical and hospitalization plan. The court determined that this plan, organized by the Group Health Association, was engaged in a business or trade and therefore was within the scope of the Sherman Act. It rejected the defense that since the plan was a cooperative, its activities were not a business. It said the case did not require the typical interstate commerce requirement because it was brought under Section 3, which applies only to the District of Columbia and the territorial possessions and does not require a showing of impact upon interstate commerce.

In this case, the United States charged in a criminal indictment that the AMA and its affiliated associations had engaged in a five-part conspiracy to obstruct the business of the prepaid health plan. The five parts consisted of the following elements: (1) restraining the prepaid plan from doing business, (2) restraining members of the prepaid plan from obtaining adequate medical care under the plan, (3) restraining doctors serving the plan in the pursuit of their calling, (4) restraining doctors not employed by the plan from practicing in the District of Columbia in pursuit of their calling, (5) restraining Washington hospitals from pursuing their own businesses.

The government contended that the defendants had conspired to coerce practicing physicians from accepting employment under the prepaid plan, to restrain practicing physicians from consulting with others employed by the plan who might desire to consult with them, and to restrain area hospitals from providing facilities for the care of patients of physicians employed by the plan.

The Supreme Court decision was something of a milestone for the application of antitrust laws in the health care industry in that the court determined for the first time that a cooperative prepaid health care plan was a business or trade within the scope of the Sherman Act. The court held that the fact that such a plan might operate as a cooperative did not remove its activities from the sphere of business. In addition, it said, the calling or occupation of the individual physicians charged as defendants was immaterial if the conspiracy had a purpose and effect to obstruct and restrain the business of the prepaid plan. Consequently, the court decided that there was no generalized exemption from the antitrust laws for the business of providing health care services. It ordered that a jury be allowed to decide whether the evidence actually showed that the organized physicians had acted to obstruct and destroy competition from the prepaid plan. However, the general charge was determined to be subject to antitrust scrutiny and enforcement.

The next major case that considered the antitrust aspects of prepaid health plans was *United States v. Oregon State Medical Society*.[54] This 1952 case differed in large part from the AMA case because the prepaid medical plan was not located in the District of Columbia, which precluded the use of Section 3 of the Sherman Act so the usual requirement of proving a substantial effect upon interstate commerce did apply.

The government charged that the Oregon State Medical Society and certain local medical societies had conspired to boycott persons who engaged in certain prepaid health programs and later had formed their own prepaid health programs and proceeded to monopolize this segment of the industry. The medical societies did not deny that at one time they had condemned the prepaid health practices and pressured individual doctors not to engage in these practices. Moreover, they had threatened expulsion from the medical societies, and one society actually had expelled several doctors for refusal to terminate contract practices.

Seven years before the lawsuit was begun, however, the societies had abandoned their boycott and organized a nonprofit corporation to provide prepaid medical, surgical, and hospital care. Subsequently, the government charged that these societies had conspired to restrain and monopolize the business of providing prepaid medical care in that state and to restrain competition among their own doctor-sponsored local plans as the statewide nonprofit corporation organized by the societies would not furnish prepaid medical care in any area already serviced by a local society's prepaid health care plan.

The Supreme Court concluded that the record showed no threat that the medical societies would revert to their boycott against other prepaid health care plans and consequently took no action against the societies on the boycott issue. As for the monopolization issues, the court similarly held that the government had failed to show a sufficient impact upon interstate commerce and, therefore, there was no jurisdiction under the Sherman Act. As noted, had this case been brought in more recent times, it is much more likely that a sufficient impact on interstate commerce could have been found.

The interstate commerce problem was avoided in a 1951 Washington state case in which a prepaid health plan charged that a county medical society and others had conspired to eliminate competition and restrain trade in contract medicine by refusing to allow plaintiff doctors to become members of the county society, by boycotting those doctors professionally, and, as in the previous case, by not permitting them to use various hospital facilities.[55]

Basing its decision on an antimonopoly section of the state constitution, the state court ruled that the defendants had conspired to eliminate competition in the practice of contract medicine. The court determined that this was improper and enjoined the defendants from excluding physicians who were practicing contract medicine in competition with the county society from becoming members of the county society. The court said the lack of membership in the county society was viewed with disfavor by community residents, patients, and other physicians, and resulted in the loss of hospital privileges, inability to be certified by the specialty boards, inability to participate in professional programs of the state and national medical associations, and failure to be called upon to act as consultants with other doctors. While the action was not based upon the federal antitrust statutes, it did rely upon the concept of joining together for the purpose of excluding another individual or individuals and thereby restraining trade.

A more recent example of similar allegations is found in *Ohio ex rel Brown v. Mahoning County Medical Society,*[56] where the Ohio state attorney general in 1976 accused two medical associations of conspiracy to prevent an HMO from operating in Youngstown and contended that such organized resistance to prevent a potential competitor from gaining access to the market constituted a *per se* violation.

The Federal Trade Commission has been particularly active in protecting prepaid health plans and in 1976 issued a consent order requiring a Washington state operator of a Blue Shield health care payment plan and an association of participating physicians to cease boycotting HMOs.[57] This decree said the defendant Medical Service Corporation was engaged in the business of establishing and administering plans in which it contracted with fee-for-service physicians to provide services to consumer subscribers. The corporation then reimbursed participating physicians for covered services to subscribers. At least 25 percent of the population of Eastern Washington subscribed to a Medical Service Corporation plan and more than 90 percent of the practicing physicians in that part of the state participated in medical service corporations. Physicians valued the status of being participating physicians and were disadvantaged by the deprivation of such status.

To meet the interstate commerce requirement, the FTC contended that substantial federal funds flowed across state lines into Eastern Washington to pay physicians' fees and encourage the development of HMOs. It charged that the Medical Service Bureau (an additional and similar defendant) and the Medical Service Corporation treated patients from other states and countries, received money from the federal government and private insurers, paid funds across state lines to other cooperating health care providers, and prescribed medicines shipped in interstate commerce, among other practices.

The FTC also charged that the Medical Service Corporation and the Medical Service Bureau individually and collectively engaged in acts that had the effect of boycotting HMOs and physicians providing services to or for HMOs. It said the Medical Service Corporation entered into provider contracts only with physicians who were or could be members of the Medical Service Bureau and refused to enter into contracts with physicians who entered into similar arrangements with other persons or organizations. The Medical Service Bureau refused membership to any physician who agreed to provide services to or for an HMO and permitted its members to become participating physicians only in the Medical Service Corporation, the FTC said. The agency also charged that the Medical Service Bureau's bylaws required that membership be granted to physicians who contracted to provide services to an HMO only if the HMO was approved by the bureau and permitted its members to become participating physicians for organizations other than the Medical Service Corporation only if the entities were approved by the bureau.

The FTC argued that the effect of these acts, practices, and methods of competition was to stabilize and interfere with the prices of physician services; to restrain competition among physicians, entry of HMOs into the physician services market, and the development of organizations offering health benefit plans using participating physician contracts; and to deprive consumers of the benefits of competition among physicians, fee-for-service medical care plans, and physician prepayment medical care plans.

The FTC decree ordered that neither of the defendants directly or indirectly enter into, adhere to, promote, or follow any course of conduct, practice, or policy, or any agreement or understanding, that discriminated against any HMO or any lawfully practicing physician, or excluded any lawfully practicing physician from being a participating physician in the Medical Service Corporation because that physician practiced medicine on other than a fee-for-service basis or was associated in any way with an HMO.

Similar allegations have been made in more recent cases,[58] and undoubtedly will continue to occur. The tension between the fee-for-service sector and the prepaid care sector is both conceptual and financial. Prepaid plans challenge and jeopardize the basic physician-patient relationship by inserting a third party as the physician's employer and a conflict between unflinching care for the patient and cost savings for the employer. They also create concern that physicians in the employ of such plans will forfeit a great deal of the professional flexibility that goes with a self-employed status. To patients and physicians, however, pre-paid plans offer certainty and stability in care and employment, respectively. These plans, existing even as a relatively small part of the total health care market, also are probably the single brightest hope for overcoming many of the economic factors that cause the fee-for-service sector to be relatively less responsive to ordinary economic incentives.

Medicaid Boycotts

Medicaid patients have been subjected to boycotts by pharmacists, dentists, and nursing homes when those providers have refused to deal with them in efforts to force rate increases. Antitrust suits have been instituted in some instances to challenge the boycotts. In one case, dentists in Ohio wrote the agency responsible for the payments stating that they were refusing to treat Medicaid patients until they were paid higher fees. The state attorney general brought an antitrust action and obtained a 1976 consent decree in which the dentists terminated their boycott and accepted the fees paid by the state for Medicaid patients.[59]

In Philadelphia, Medicaid patients sued in 1978, claiming they had been denied access to skilled nursing facilities through a conspiracy by nursing homes to increase prices.[60] The plaintiffs alleged that the defendants had agreed to refuse Medicaid patients until a rate increase was granted. The court refused to grant the defendants' motion to dismiss for failure to state a claim. Nursing home operators in other states have been faced with similar antitrust suits when they have sought to boycott Medicaid patients.[61]

The New York attorney general similarly filed an antitrust action in 1978 against a pharmaceutical society that advocated a Medicaid boycott, and the state obtained an injunction.[62] The court found that the society's conduct through the boycott unreasonably restrained trade. The injunction provided that society members could not refrain from dispensing drugs to Medicaid patients and could not withdraw from the Medicaid program for a specified period of time.

Other Boycotts

Perhaps the most dramatic medical boycott occurred in California when physicians, distressed about malpractice insurance rates, jointly stopped working (often referred to as a physicians' "strike") to protest rate increases in malpractice coverage and to draw attention to their requests that the state legislature pass certain legal reform measures to help alleviate the problems. Although no antitrust actions were instituted to challenge this joint refusal to work, it has been reported that an action was being prepared when the physicians terminated the "strike."[63] Such an action undoubtedly would have raised novel legal issues, as the physicians essentially were using a group boycott against patients and hospitals to influence legislative action, but with no anticompetitive motive against the parties who actually were subjected to the boycott. As the boycott was not horizontal in nature (*i.e.*, one group of competitors was not boycotting other competitors), it is unlikely the conduct would amount to a *per se* offense. The reasonableness of the conduct certainly is questionable, however, and a concerted refusal to deal with patients, and particularly with hospitals, that had the foreseeable consequence of severely damaging the business of many hospitals, could well be held to constitute an unreasonable restraint of trade.

Physicians participating in such a politically oriented boycott might contend, quite properly, that the antitrust laws have been held inapplicable to political activity. The conduct in this instance may have been primarily political in motive, but it was only indirectly political in effect. To pursue political ends through direct restraints of trade would appear, at best, to jeopardize the antitrust exemptions and immunities otherwise available for those engaged in, or attempting to influence, political processes, although other recent developments indicate some latitude may continue to be allowed to those who utilize the boycott mechanism to effect political ends.[64] It also is important to note, in this context, that the antitrust exemptions available for bona fide labor disputes do not extend to joint work-stoppage agreements among persons in business who are not under the supervision of an organized union.

In a more typical situation, the Federal Trade Commission in 1978 charged two groups of Indiana dentists with restricting the efforts of health insurers to maintain the cost of dental care.[65] The FTC issued a complaint against one of the associations, charging that the dental health care programs provided for a decision on benefits in advance of treatment, which limited the insurance to the least expensive treatment determined by standard dental procedures. The reason for the requirement of the least expensive method was to hold the cost of dental care to its minimum level. Dentists were required to furnish patients' x-rays to insurance companies for the system to operate efficiently.

The association, in an apparent effort to inhibit the activities of the health insurers, organized its members to refuse to submit patient x-rays so insurance benefits could not be determined, encouraged dentists not to serve as consultants to insurance companies, issued guidelines to members on procedures for dealing with dental health insurance programs, and urged its members to agree not to compete with other dentists in dealing with insurance plans. The result of these efforts was potentially adverse to dental care cost control for consumers, prevented consumers from obtaining a second dentist's opinion, restrained competition among dentists, and limited the number of dentists who would cooperate with dental insurance plans. The FTC therefore filed an action to prohibit the association from engaging in any of those challenged activities.

While technically not a case involving an official association, but rather a group of physicians in a geographic area who controlled the market for obstetric-gynecological services, a Florida women's health center that provided first trimester elective abortions brought suit in 1976 against those physicians, charging they had engaged in a conspiracy or a combination that constituted a boycott of the health center's clinic in violation of federal and state antitrust laws.[66] The center also alleged that the doctors monopolized the market for providing women's health and abortion services. The case highlights the potential actions that may arise when a group of physicians, even without the status of a trade association,[67] combines to prevent new competition in their market. While the district court granted summary judgment for the defendants on all counts, the appellate court in 1978 reversed the decision,[68] as a result of which the case could proceed to trial.

STANDARDIZATION AND QUALITY STANDARDS

The activities historically characteristic of trade associations include setting standards and promoting standardization of the products of the trade. Typically, an association will approve products that meet its standards, a process not unlike accreditation or certification. Understandably, the antitrust problems also are similar: an association must set and administer product standards in a reasonable manner, one not calculated to discriminate against competitors.[69]

Standardization is not itself illegal, and the courts and the FTC recognize that standardization can have beneficial and procompetitive effects.[70] Although standardization is commonly the work of governmental regulatory agencies,[71] a trade association typically works closely with an agency developing product standards. In fact, the association may have petitioned for and prompted the government's standard setting.[72]

Involvement with a government agency will not, however, in itself insulate an association from antitrust liability. Regardless of whether the standards bear the government's imprimatur, if an association influences the development of governmental standards it may be liable for abuse of that influence. Thus, in one case, a trade association of plywood manufacturers had been the primary impetus for the adoption of product standards by the Department of Commerce and had continued to contribute to subsequent revision of those standards. A nonmember manufacturer of the product with a new, as yet unapproved, process was unable to sell his products without certification. The manufacturer sued the association, alleging that the association was responsible for the Commerce Department's failure to amend its standards to accept the new process. The court agreed with the manufacturer's contention that the association was responsible not only for its own set of standards, but also for the government's. The court found, however, that the association was not liable under the antitrust laws because it had acted reasonably in its testing of the new process.[73]

Associations that grant "seals of approval" must award them on an objective basis, with reasonable testing procedures.[74] For example, associations may not discriminate against the products of competitors of their members[75] or against the products of foreign manufacturers,[76] and associations that publish product standards must not enforce them themselves; compliance should be voluntary.[77]

The Federal Trade Commission has proposed a rule for regulating "standards developers, certifiers, and persons who reference standards or certification in the marketing of products."[78] The proposal would establish minimum procedural standards for standard making, establishing and emphasizing a right of the public to participate in the standard-making process, and would establish basic criteria for the substance of standards that would be the measure by which those that are challenged as unfair, deceptive, or anticompetitive would be judged.

The proposed rule also would regulate the standards of certifiers. For example, the proposal would require a certifier to require a seller using its seal of approval to disclose certain specific information, such as the substance of the certification as it related to the product. The rule also would prohibit basing certification on factors such as "a producer's trade association membership, size of the producer, product origin and whether a product is intended for retrofit rather than installation as original equipment."[79] While quite comprehensive, the proposed rule would not affect standards of professional competence and other "nonproduct standards."[80]

Standardization of services or products under certain circumstances also may be a vehicle for unlawful price fixing, a *per se* offense under the Sherman Act.[81] For example, when associated with the sharing of price information, product standardization may be further evidence of the probability of price fixing, on the ground that having standardized products makes it easier for producers of a good to understand the pricing policies of their competitors.[82]

An association also may be liable for price fixing through product standardization even though the affected amount was not the price of the product of the members of the association. In *National Macaroni Manufacturers Association v. Federal Trade Commission*,[83] for example, members of a trade association, while not coordinating their own prices or otherwise limiting their competition, agreed to market a lower quality product to prolong short supplies of the essential ingredient of the high quality product, and thus stabilize the price of the ingredient. The court held that the agreement constituted unlawful fixing of the price of the ingredient.

In health care trade associations and professional societies, quality standards are most relevant with respect to certification of health care professionals.[84] The associations usually dictate the standards their members are to follow, and hospitals sometimes adopt such policies. With increasing governmental regulation of the health care industry, some of the functions traditionally carried out by trade associations may transfer to a governmental agency, thus eliminating some of this concern

For patients, the importance of setting high standards and maintaining quality in the industry should not be underestimated. As more regulations are adopted, the associations are likely to be confronted with antitrust suits, either for setting unfair standards or for discrimination against nonmembers. Price fixing also is an obvious possibility. By standardizing practices within an industry, those providing services will understand better the pricing policies of their competitors.

DETERMINING AND SUGGESTING FEES

The most characteristic attribute of monopoly power is the power to set prices regardless of market forces, and perhaps the most characteristic violation of the antitrust laws is an agreement to fix prices. A price-fixing agreement among competitors is a *per se* violation of Section 1 of the Sherman Act and as such is unlawful regardless of any beneficial purposes it serves.[85] An agreement to fix prices similarly is not made lawful because the price fixed is "reasonable."[86]

Because of this long reach of the *per se* rule against price fixing, it is rare for an association to dictate openly, or even to suggest, prices to its members. Where associations have done so, the price-fixing orders generally have been held unlawful,[87] even when the members of the group typically discounted from the association's suggested list prices when making sales, and despite the continued existence, after the price fixing, of other open avenues of competition.[88]

Thus, as a result of the *per se* rule, the most common instances of overt price fixing by trade groups have arisen in the context of associations of professionals, such as lawyers and doctors, who for many years enjoyed immunity from the Sherman Act since their businesses were not considered "trade or commerce." Under this protective umbrella, professional associations commonly published schedules of minimum fees and codes of ethics restricting competition by, among other things, price.[89] However, the Supreme Court has steadily expanded the definition of "trade" as used in the Sherman Act,[90] and, in the landmark case of *Goldfarb v. Virginia State Bar*,[91] the court held that Congress had not intended to exclude the learned professions from the purview of the Sherman Act. Therefore, a bar association that had published a set of minimum fees for legal services (real estate title searches, in this case) and had enforced the fee schedules with a code of ethics and the threat of discipline, had fixed prices in violation of the Sherman Act. The court noted that the minimum fee schedules of a professional association were especially suspect when the group had the exclusive power to authorize the practice of a profession, and where the services subject to the fixed prices were services necessary to a transaction.[92]

Nevertheless, the *Goldfarb* decision did not shut the door completely on special treatment of the professions under the antitrust laws. In a suggestive footnote, the court stated:

> [I]t would be unrealistic to view the practice of professions as interchangable with other business activities, and automatically to apply to the professions antitrust concepts which originated in other areas. The public service aspect, and other features of the profession may require that particular practice, which could properly be viewed as a violation of the Sherman Act in another context, be treated differently.[93]

However, when the National Society of Professional Engineers relied upon this footnote in arguing that its prohibition against competitive bidding for engineering services was lawful as a necessary professional ethical canon adopted to protect the public safety from inferior engineering work, which it contended would occur in the event competitive bidding were allowed, the Supreme Court was unpersuaded.[94] In the words of the court:

> We are faced with a contention that a total ban on competitive bidding is necessary because otherwise engineers will be tempted to submit deceptively low bids. Certainly the problem of professional deception is a proper subject of an ethical canon. But once again, the equation of competition with deception, like the similar equation with safety hazards, is simply too broad; we may assume that competition is not entirely conducive to ethical behavior, but that is not a reason, cognizable under the Sherman Act, for doing away with competition.[95]

It is similarly reasonable to believe that the *Goldfarb* and *National Society of Engineers* rules are applicable to the medical professions.[96]

Fee Setting and Influencing by Health Service Sellers

What constitutes price fixing in the health care industry, especially with regard to professional fees, is a disputed subject. While the overt or thinly disguised setting of minimum fees by professional associations is certainly unlawful in the wake of *Goldfarb*, many other professional association practices that indirectly affect prices have not been tested fully.

As evidenced by *Goldfarb* and *National Society of Engineers*, ethical guidelines promulgated by professional societies may reflect unlawful restrictions on price competition, and the FTC has attacked ethical guidelines in the health care industry as price fixing.

For instance, in a 1978 case the FTC sued the American Society of Anesthesiologists, contending that its guidelines required that anesthesiologists be compensated only on a fee-for-service basis, thus prohibiting society members from practicing as salaried employees of entities such as hospitals. The FTC charged that these restrictions on compensation deprived consumers of the benefits of this form of competition among anesthesiologists. The society entered into a consent decree[97] in which it agreed not to restrain or impede anesthesiologists from practicing on other than a fee-for-service basis and not to consider the compensation arrangements of member physicians to be matters of professional ethics.

Trade associations, particularly professional groups, have commonly promulgated ethical standards for the advertisements and promotional activities of their members. While there is some room under the antitrust laws for industry self-regulation, restrictions on advertising—particularly outright prohibitions on advertising by professionals—have been attacked as anticompetitive in recent years. The leading case on this subject is *Bates v. State Bar of Arizona*,[98] where the Supreme Court in a 1977 decision held that the First Amendment prevented the Supreme Court of Arizona, as part of its regulation of the state bar, from prohibiting advertising by lawyers. The high court limited regulation of attorney advertising to reasonable restrictions on time, place, and manner, as well as prohibitions of advertisements that were false or misleading.

While the decision rested on the First Amendment rather than the antitrust laws, since the challenged restrictions fell within the state action exemption, it is reasonable to assume that, absent state action, an agreement among competitors to refrain from advertising would be an unreasonable restraint of trade as it could eliminate an important form of competition. Unless the agreement was reasonable under the circumstances, it would be unlawful.[99] Thus, an FTC administrative law judge ruled in 1978 that the ban on physician advertising by the American Medical Association was an unfair method of competition in violation of Section 5 of the Federal Trade Commission Act because, according to the FTC complaint, it "stabilized, fixed or otherwise interfered with" the prices of physicians' services.[100]

In response to the expansion of both the antitrust laws and the First Amendment into the realm of professional advertising, several professional groups have acted to bring their codes of ethics into compliance with recent decisions. For instance, the American Physical Therapy Association in 1978 amended its code of ethics to permit advertising,[101] and the American Osteopathic Association referred the issue of member advertising to its committee on ethics.[102] Presumably, other associations either are conforming with new perceptions of allowable standards or consciously choosing to risk litigation.

Peer Review Procedures

Insurance companies or the government, through programs such as Medicare and Medicaid, now pay for a large percentage of health care services. As the typical health care customer has become a large-scale institution rather than an individual, there has been the perception of a tendency to develop uniform pricing policies for health care services. The plans may depend on the cooperation of trade and professional groups, which may review the performance of practitioners and then devise fee standards for particular procedures. Such peer review systems thus may tend to fix prices.

In *Bartholomew v. Virginia Chiropractors Association, Inc.*,[103] individual chiropractors challenged the peer review procedure used by health insurance carriers in conjunction with the Virginia Chiropractors Association and the American Chiropractic Association. The carriers' contract with insured individuals and groups limited reimbursement to usual and customary charges for necessary health care services, and the chiropractic peer review committee determined the usual and customary fees for chiropractic services. The plaintiffs in *Bartholomew* charged that the associations and the carriers had set maximum compensation levels that were not adequate compensation for the services the plaintiffs provided.[104] While the court did not reach the merits,[105] it indicated that if the facts were as alleged, the associations and carriers had coerced the plaintiffs unlawfully to charge according to the determinations of the peer review committees.[106]

While avoiding specifying fees, medical societies have promoted uniformity among the fee-setting policies of health care providers by using "relative value scales"—lists of medical procedures setting comparative numerical values for various procedures performed and/or services rendered by physicians and other health care providers. A relative value scale provides comparable value for varying medical procedures. For example, a schedule might provide that setting a broken leg should cost twice as much as closing a small wound with stitches.

The FTC has entered into a number of consent decrees with medical societies prohibiting them from engaging in relative value scale or study activities. In one such consent order, agreed to by the American College of Radiology, the FTC commented:

> Adherence to a relative value scale freezes the relationship among fees for different procedures. For instance, even where physicians individually set conversion factors, if they follow a relative value scale that assigns a Procedure "A" three times the number of units as Procedure "B", Procedure "A" will always be three times as costly as Procedure "B" . . .
> In addition publication of a relative value scale makes it convenient

for physicians to fix prices across the board merely by agreeing to a uniform conversion. . . .[107]

DETERMINING AND SUGGESTING PRICES PAID

The *per se* rule against price fixing is not restricted to agreements among sellers of goods or services, but embraces buyers as well. Thus, in the leading case of *Mandeville Island Farms, Inc. v. American Crystal Sugar Co.,*[108] the Supreme Court in 1948 proscribed an arrangement whereby refiners of sugar beets agreed on the prices they would pay sugar beet producers.[109] This type of problem might arise most typically for health providers in the context of conduct influencing salary levels or the prices paid for various commodities used in running an institution.

DISSEMINATION OF STATISTICAL INFORMATION

While an agreement is a necessary element of a conspiracy to violate the Sherman Act,[110] an agreement to conspire to fix prices need not be overt. A conspiracy may be inferred from the relationships and conduct between or among competitors or trading partners, even if they are not in direct communication,[111] if the conduct produces price stability, particularly if there is no indication of a lawful purpose. While competitors may establish a relationship for lawful purposes, within such a combination a conspiracy to restrain trade unlawfully may be found, implied even by apparently lawful activities.[112] As a cooperative combination of competitors, a trade association thus may provide a framework for implications of unlawful implied conspiracies in restraint of trade.

An association must be careful that its lawful cooperative activities do not lead to a decline in price competition because such an effect may imply an agreement to fix prices. There are many typical association activities that, despite the absence of an overt agreement, may imply price fixing. Most often suspect are agreements by members to have the association collect and disseminate prices, or statistical information relevant to prices, such as stocks on hand, total orders, and—perhaps most suggestive of price fixing—forecasts of future price activity. The compilation of statistical data commonly is one of the most significant activities of a trade or professional association, and the activity may serve many beneficial and procompetitive purposes. Therefore, the threshold point at which information gathering becomes an agreement to fix prices is important.

The leading cases on statistical reporting particularly emphasize the importance of the intent of the proponents of a plan to compile and disseminate the data, and consider other factors relevant to whether a statistical reporting program is reasonable under the circumstances. Thus, the lawfulness of such a plan depends on the presence or absence of various factors that indicate whether the agreement to compile and disseminate statistics is a conspiracy to limit price competition.

One important factor is the voluntariness of the plan. For example, where members agreed to send the association all their price lists and, on a daily basis, records of any deviations from those prices, and further agreed to deposit funds with the association that would be forfeited for not complying with the scheme, the provisions for the compilation of price statistics and dissemination of them among the parties to the agreement were held to be unlawful.[113] In comparison, evidence that recipients of distributed list price information regularly made off-list sales has indicated that there was no intent to fix prices by disseminating the information.[114] Consequently, programs for statistic compilation and reporting should not include procedures for review and evaluation of a participant's compliance with the plan.

Statistical reporting services of associations also should be open to nonmembers. As free access to information is procompetitive, the courts favor open reporting of statistics. As Justice Oliver Wendell Holmes stated in 1921, "I should have thought that the ideal of commerce was an intelligent interchange made with full knowledge of the facts as a basis for a forecast of the future on both sides."[115] The example here is the open market or exchange, where dealers assemble and buy and sell openly.[116]

Knowledge of industry conditions translates into economic power, so secret reporting implies that the purpose of the data gathering is to give the sector of the industry sharing the statistics a particular advantage. Thus, in a case where the Sugar Institute,[117] an association of sugar refiners, compiled statistics on varying matters, including total production and deliveries, but made only some of the information available to customers, the trial court found that the information withheld from the purchasing trade was what was meaningful to a customer, while the material disseminated outside the association was valueless, or even misleading, for any individual customer. Therefore, "by collecting and circulating only among themselves that information, defendants obtained an unfair advantage with respect to purchasers and effected an unreasonable restraint."[118] In contrast, open statistical reporting programs have been upheld as procompetitive, even when the statistics included price information.[119]

The reporting of price statistics is best restricted to data from past transactions to avoid implying "forecasting." However, even if a price reporting plan formally encompasses only past transactions, it still may indicate a forecasting and price influencing plan if it includes the collection and dissemination of other information not necessarily pertaining directly to prices. Thus, where an association collected not only past prices but also inquired as to the expectations of its members as to future production and their views on upcoming market conditions, the Supreme Court found that the plan suggested an attempt to harmonize prices.[120] It should be noted that forecasting is not itself unlawful but it does aid prosecutions for price fixing by assisting plaintiffs and prosecutors in creating the inference of an agreement to abide by the forecasts.

The nature of the industry and its products or services also is relevant to whether a statistics reporting plan constitutes a conspiracy to fix prices. In industries where a product is standardized, the dissemination of price statistics is more likely to indicate price fixing than in industries characterized by unstandardized or made-to-order products, since in industries with standardized products it is relatively easy to evaluate the pricing policies of one's competitors.[121] Thus, if competitors market a commodity such as sugar, that by its nature restricts them to competition by price, dissemination of information relating to price only among the competitors will be suspect.[122] In seeming contrast, however, price fixing is more likely to be inferred from price reporting in industries where customers can shop for prices, as opposed to industries characterized by exclusive supply contracts, where prices are determined by long-term contracts.[123] If a customer and a seller are locked in a long-term contract, the fact that the seller and its competitors share price information will have little impact on the customer's deal.

In the health care industry, the antitrust problems created by data dissemination are relevant with respect to relative value studies (discussed earlier) as examples of price fixing.[124] The publication of relative value scales entails data compilation and the scales themselves are forms of statistical summaries. The information they contain is important to the formulation of health care fiscal policy and to a rational understanding of the cost structure of the industry. Yet, as noted, relative value scales may affect price. To protect the information-gathering role of health care trade and professional associations, the consent decrees prohibiting the use of relative value scales to fix prices, entered into by and between the FTC and medical societies, have not prohibited the groups from furnishing testimony, or whatever information may be requested, to government entities or others involved in paying for health services. For example, the consent decree[125] in *United States v. Illinois Podiatry Society, Inc.* provided:

> Nothing in this Final Judgment shall prohibit defendants or its Appeals, Controls, and Review Commission from furnishing testimony or information to any third party directly engaged in the provision, reimbursement, indemnification or prepayment of the costs of health services; to the extent, however, that such information or testimony may bear directly or indirectly on compensation levels for podiatric services or procedures it shall be limited to information or testimony derived solely from the professional experience of the individual members of defendant without reference to any relative value study or similar compilation. . . .[126]

While at one time the Supreme Court considered a *per se* rule against the sharing of price information by competitors, it appears now to have returned to a reasonableness standard. In 1969, in *United States v. Container Corporation of America*,[127] the possibility of a *per se* rule arose because the court found that even an unsystematic and informal process of exchanging price information among the major competitors in an industry constituted price fixing when it "seemed to have the effect of keeping prices within a fairly narrow ambit."[128] Although the court included in its opinion the statement that "[p]rice is too critical, too sensitive a control to allow it to be used even in an informal manner to restrain competition,"[129] it did not explicitly state a *per se* rule against the exchange of price information, and one justice expressed his understanding that the decision had not established such a rule.[130] The court resolved the question six years later, when it adopted this justice's view and stated that "the dissemination of price information is not itself a *per se* violation of the Sherman Act."[131] Thus, the courts will continue to apply to statistic dissemination cases the factors discussed above and further identified in early cases such as *American Column and Lumber*,[132] *Sugar Institute*,[133] and *Linseed Oil*.[134]

Similarly, courts have used a multifactor reasoning process to permit associations to compile and disseminate information regarding the credit of their members' customers, even though the distribution of a bad credit report might lead to a boycott. A common activity of associations, particularly those of businesses regularly selling products or services to specific and common groups of customers, is to compile and to distribute credit reports on the buyers. These reports undoubtedly discourage business with delinquent customers and might be considered implied boycotts. In addition, credit is an aspect of price, and thus the dissemination of credit information logically might be scrutinized as dissemination of price information.

Nevertheless, credit reporting services have been upheld if necessary to prevent fraud so long as there is no agreement for mandatory restrictions on trading with delinquent customers.[135] As with determining prices, an individual decision not to advance credit to a customer does not by itself violate the antitrust laws since this type of violation generally requires an agreement, unless the conduct amounts to actual or attempted monopolization.

COOPERATIVE BUYING AND SELLING AND DIVISION OF MARKETS

Because of the cost advantages of buying in large lots and the economies of scale often available when services are provided to different entities from a central source, and because members of trade associations typically have similar needs for goods and services, a natural activity of these associations has been cooperative buying for their members. However, while permissible, cooperative buying poses problems under the Robinson-Patman Act, which under certain conditions prohibits the granting or receiving of "discriminatory" prices. If membership in the buying cooperative is restricted, the cooperative buying program also may violate the Sherman Act, particularly if it tends to create a division of markets or confer monopolistic powers upon its members.

The Robinson-Patman Act[136] is discussed in detail in Chapter 8. Briefly stated, however, that act differs markedly from other antitrust laws in that, instead of outlawing price stability, it requires it under certain circumstances. Assuming jurisdictional and procedural requirements to invoke the act are met, it generally forbids a seller to grant lower prices to a buyer, or a buyer to accept lower prices from a seller, solely on the ground that the buyer purchases a large volume of goods. Lower prices to large purchasers may reflect legally only actual lower costs of processing larger orders or a good faith attempt to meet the prices of competitors.[137]

Since the "meeting competition" defense generally is limited to a "defensive" meeting of a competitor's price by an individual seller,[138] for practical purposes the defense more relevant to the conduct of a buying cooperative (which, as a purchaser, may be liable along with the seller under the act) is to show that the lower prices it pays are justified by reduced costs to the seller. To show that the seller has savings to pass through to a buying cooperative, it is necessary that the latter do more than merely tabulate its members' purchases. A buying cooperative must be more than a mere shell within which individual member-buyers place their orders directly with and receive delivery directly from the seller. Under such circumstances, the FTC and the courts frequently have found quantity discounts to violate the Robinson-Patman Act.[139] In contrast, when a buying cooperative performs significant functions such as warehousing a stock of goods, the quantity discount has been approved as reflective of cost savings.[140] In such a case, the cooperative acts as a wholesaler and deserves a "wholesale" price. It thus is important that a buying cooperative be as active as possible, and as independent as possible from its members.

Buying cooperatives also may raise antitrust problems as unlawful agreements to divide markets horizontally, or as unlawful boycotts, if membership requirements are restrictive. In *United States v. Topco Associates, Inc.*,[141] the Supreme Court held that a cooperative buying association of small and medium-sized regional supermarket chains violated Section 1 of the Sherman Act by restricting membership so as to avoid competition between members operating in the same geographic areas. The association argued that the restriction was necessary to its effectiveness and that any anticompetitive effects of its restrictions were outweighed by the procompetitive effects of enabling its members to compete effectively against large, national supermarket chains. The court, however, rejected this argument on the ground that a horizontal division of markets was a *per se* violation of the Act and therefore that reasonableness, assuming the arrangement was reasonable, was irrelevant.[142] It thus appears that, because of the direct economic significance of cooperative buying, the standards for openness of membership in associations with cooperative buying programs are higher than for other membership benefits, since reasonable exclusions in other contexts are allowed.[143] Alternatively, all geographic restrictions on membership where membership has some value may be unlawful.[144]

Providers that choose to associate together in cooperative buying or shared service organizations, where the organization takes the form of an association as opposed to a corporate joint venture that might be analyzed under the antimerger laws, should be particularly wary not to establish membership requirements that unnecessarily disadvantage excluded competitors. In addition, if the association becomes large enough to acquire monopoly power as a purchaser (monopsony), the conduct might well be characterized as monopolization and scrutinized under Section 2 of the Sherman Act. Simply forming an association to create bargaining and purchasing power sufficient to reduce the cost of purchased goods, however, is not in itself illegal and, if used properly, could be a significant aid in the effort to curb cost increases.

Shared service organizations of this sort also should be cautious to avoid packaging their functions in a manner that may constitute the tying of separable products and services. For example, where a shared service organization provides a group purchasing function for member institutions, it may be entirely unnecessary and even unreasonable to compel members to participate in the group buying of multiple products or services. Where the organization allows members to participate in only the group purchases they desire, it can avoid being charged with using its market power in some functions to tie in the requirement of participating in other functions and thus avoid a very real possibility of violating Section 1 of the Sherman Act or Section 3 of the Clayton Act.

LOBBYING

A final characteristic function of a trade or professional association is promoting the views of its members on public matters affecting their business through lobbying and similar activities. While lobbying itself is considered in more detail in Chapter 3, it is of value to examine briefly the antitrust treatment of lobbying by trade associations.

Associations frequently lobby to ensure that their arguments are heard above those of competitors and, in effect, to restrain the trade of competitors. Consequently, an association's efforts to advance the cause of its members through political action may injure the business of competitors. Nevertheless, all but the most extraordinary efforts of an association to advance the interests of its members through political action or the petitioning of governmental authorities are insulated from antitrust liability under the doctrine of *Eastern Railroad Presidents Conference v. Noerr Motor Freight, Inc.,*[145] in which the Supreme Court subordinated the antitrust laws to the rights to associate and to petition the government. The court ruled that Congress had not enacted the Sherman Act to regulate political activity, and that the right of the people to associate and present their views on matters of public interest to the government overrode any anticompetitive effects of such an association.[146]

The court did not, however, completely immunize political action from the antitrust laws. It left open the possibility that "[t]here may be situations in which a publicity campaign, ostensibly directed toward influencing governmental action, is a mere sham to cover what is actually nothing more than an attempt to interfere directly with the business relationships of a competitor and the application of the Sherman Act would be justified."[147] In *California Motor Transport Co. v. Trucking Unlimited,*[148] the court seized on this language to allow a group of trucking companies to sue a group of competing truckers on the ground that the defendants had conspired to abuse judicial and administrative procedures to prevent the plaintiffs from being awarded operating rights. Of particular importance to the court was the plaintiffs' allegation that the defendants were not interested in influencing public officials but only in preventing the plaintiffs from doing so, thereby "to usurp [the] . . . decision-making process."[149]

The mere fact that an association performs lobbying functions, however, will not shelter it from other antitrust scrutiny. Where, for example, membership in a lobbying oriented association becomes a virtual economic necessity, membership rules must be reasonable and not calculated for anticompetitive ends, just as with any other economically significant association.

NOTES

1. *Veizaga v. Nat'l Bd. for Respiratory Therapy*, 1977—1 Trade Cases (CCH) ¶ 61,274 (N.D. Ill. 1977).

2. *See, e.g., United States v. Allied Florists Ass'n of Illinois*, 1953 Trade Cases ¶ 67,433 (N.D. Ill. 1953) (consent decree provided, *inter alia*, that defendant "[a]dmit to its membership any retail florist, grower or wholesaler on non-discriminatory terms and conditions").

3. *See, e.g., United States v. Florists' Telegraph Delivery Ass'n*, 1956 Trade Cases ¶ 68,367 (E.D. Mich. 1956) (consent decree prohibited defendant from "[e]xcluding from membership . . . any florist for the reason that such florist is a member or proposes to become a member of any other wire association").

4. *See, Deesen v. Professional Golfers' Ass'n of America*, 158 F.2d 165 (9th Cir. 1966), where a professional golfer alleged that defendant's rules and regulations governing eligibility for its tournaments unreasonably restrained his business. The court found that it was reasonable for defendants to enforce criteria restricting access to the tournament because its purpose, "to insure that professional golf tournaments [were] not bogged down with great numbers of players of inferior ability," was reasonable. 358 F.2d at 170. *See also, United States v. Southern Wholesale Grocers' Ass'n*, 207 F.

434, 439–40 (N.D. Ala. 1913) (an association of wholesale grocers could demand of its members that they refrain from retail sales, since "otherwise [it would] have been impossible to maintain an association composed only of the wholesale grocers . . ."); *Compare, American Fed'n of Tobacco Growers, Inc. v. Neal*, 183 F.2d 869, 872 (4th Cir. 1950) (a board of trade with monopoly control over local commerce in tobacco could not deny membership on the ground that applicant's warehouse was located outside city limits).

5. *See Willner v. Comm. on Character and Fitness*, 373 U.S. 96, 83 S.Ct. 1175 (1963) (withholding of a license to practice law requires a hearing on the charges filed against the applicant); *Silver v. New York Stock Exchange*, 373 U.S. 341, 83 S.Ct. 1246 (1963) (a stock exchange and its members could not terminate access to an essential service that the exchange provided without procedural safeguards such as notice and a hearing.); *Compare, Tropic Film Corp. v. Paramount Pictures Corp.*, 319 F.Supp. 1247, 1249 (S.D. N.Y. 1970) (less rigorous procedures required when restricted benefit is not essential).

6. *Associated Press v. United States*, 326 U.S. 1, 65 S.Ct. 1416 (1945).

7. Freedom of Association is protected by the due process clause of the Fourteenth Amendment to the United States Constitution. *See NAACP v. Alabama*, 357 U.S. 449 (1958).

8. *Manok v. Southeast Dist. Bowling Ass'n*, 306 F.Supp. 1215, 1221 (C.D. Cal. 1969).

9. *See, e.g., Deesen v. Professional Golfers' Ass'n of America, supra,* note *4.*

10. *See* Chapter 6 on medical staff privileges.

11. *Higgins v. Am. Soc'y of Clinical Pathologists*, 51 N.J. 191, 238 A.2d 665 (1968); *Schooler v. Tarrant County Medical Soc'y*, 457 S.W. 2d 644 (Tex. Civ. App. 1970); *Washington Osteopathic Medical Ass'n v. King County Medical Serv. Corp.*, 78 Wash.2d 577, 478 P.2d 228 (1970); *Pinsker v. Pacific Coast Soc'y of Orthodontists*, 12 Cal. 3d 541, 116 Cal.Rptr. 245 (1974); *Pima County Medical Soc'y v. Felland*, 115 Ariz. 311, 565 P.2d 188 (1977).

12. The allegation was that the American Dental Ass'n membership requirement created an anticompetitive tying arrangement by limiting participation in the state and local associations to ADA members.

13. *Boddicker v. Arizona State Dental Ass'n*, 549 F.2d 626 (9th Cir.), *cert. denied*, 434 U.S. 825 (1977).

14. 421 U.S. 773, 95 S.Ct. 2004 (1975). *See* Chapter 1.

15. 428 U.S. 579, 96 S.Ct. 3110 (1976).

16. *Marjorie Webster Junior College, Inc. v. Middle States Ass'n of Colleges and Secondary Schools, Inc.*, 432 F.2d 650 (D.C. Cir. 1969) (held, reasonable to deny membership in an association of educational institutions, and thus accreditation, to a for-profit school).

17. *Id.*, at 654.

18. *See* Chapter 1 on state action.

19. *See* Chapter 1 on boycotts.

20. *Cypress v. Newport News General & Nonsectarian Hosp. Ass'n*, 375 F.2d 648 (4th Cir. 1967); *Hawkins v. North Carolina Dental Soc'y*, 355 F.2d 718 (4th Cir. 1966); *Aasum v. Good Samaritan Hosp.*, 542 F.2d 792 (9th Cir. 1976); *Bell v. Georgia Dental Ass'n*, 231 F.Supp. 279 (N.D. Ga. 1964); *Rao v. Bd. of County Commissioners*, 80 Wash.2d 695, 497 P.2d 591 (1972).

21. *See, e.g., United States Dental Inst. v. Am. Ass'n of Orthodontists*, 396 F.Supp. 565 (N.D. Ill. 1975) (private dental school and general practitioner dentists action against association which grants certification for orthodontists).

22. *Veizaga v. Nat'l Bd. for Respiratory Therapy*, 1977—1 Trade Cases (CCH) ¶ 61,274 (N.D. Ill. 1977).

23. Refusal to deal is an antitrust concept that sometimes signifies a situation different from a classic boycott in which parties prevent trade with a party, but it often is used as a synonym for a boycott.

24. To state a cause of action for attempted monopolization, a plaintiff is required to show that the defendant had the specific intent to gain a monopoly and that a dangerous probability of its success exists.

25. 582 F.2d 277 (3d Cir. 1978).

26. *Id.*, at 286.

27. *See, e.g., Salter v. New York State Psychological Ass'n*, 14 N.Y.2d 100, 248 N.Y.S.2d 867 (1964); *New York State Osteopathic Soc'y, Inc. v. Allen*, 26 N.Y.2d 20, 308 N.Y.S.2d 342 (1970); *Pinsker v. Pacific Coast Soc'y of Orthodontists*, 12 Cal.3d 541, 116 Cal.Rptr. 245, 526 P.2d 253 (1974).

28. *United States Dental Inst. v. Am. Ass'n of Orthodontists*, 396 F.Supp. 565 (N.D. Ill. 1975).

29. *Id.*, at 580.

30. Staff privilege denials are discussed in detail in Chapter 6.

31. 34 N.J. 582, 170 A.2d 791, 89 ALR 2d 952 (1961).

32. 170 A.2d at 799, 89 ALR 2d at 963.

33. *Greisman v. Newcomb Hosp.*, 40 N.J. 389, 192 A.2d 817 (1963).

34. *Kurk v. Medical Soc'y of County of Queens, Inc.*, 24 A.D.2d 897, 264 N.Y.S.2d 859 (1965).

35. *Pima County Medical Soc'y v. Felland*, 115 Ariz. 311, 565 P.2d 188 (1977).

36. *Spears Free Clinic and Hosp. v. Cleere*, 197 F.2d 125 (10th Cir. 1952).

37. *See* Chapter 1.

38. *Ballard v. Blue Shield of Southern W. Virginia, Inc.*, 543 F.2d 1075 (4th Cir. 1976).

39. *New Jersey Chiropractic Soc'y v. Radiological Soc'y of N.J.*, 1978–1 Trade Cases (CCH) ¶ 61,894.

40. The question of whether a person has standing can be phrased also as whether a person may bring the action. Only certain individuals, groups, or corporations are permitted to bring actions.

41. *Alabama Optometric Assn. v. Alabama State Bd. of Health*, 379 F.Supp. 1332 (M.D. Ala. 1974).

42. 269 F.2d 167 (8th Cir. 1959).

43. *Cowen v. New York Stock Exchange*, 256 F. Supp. 462 (N.D. N.Y. 1966), *aff'd*, 371 F.2d 661 (2d Cir. 1967). *See also, Molinas v. Nat'l Basketball Ass'n*, 190 F.Supp. 241 (S.D.N.Y. 1961) (held, a professional basketball player may be suspended indefinitely by a basketball league for gambling in violation of his contract without a hearing, since the offense was sufficiently serious and was otherwise proved or admitted).

44. If the rules are unreasonable, enforcement will violate the antitrust laws. *See Fashion Originators Guild of Am. v. Federal Trade Commission*, 312 U.S. 457, 61 S.Ct. 703 (1941).

45. *See e.g., McCreery Angus Farms v. American Angus Ass'n*, 379 F.Supp. 1008, 1019 (S.D. Ill. 1974); *Cowen v. New York Stock Exchange, supra*, note 43, 371 F.2d at 663–64.

46. *Blalock v. Ladies Professional Golf Ass'n*, 359 F.Supp. 1260 (N.D. Ga. 1973).

47. *Firestone v. First Dist. Dental Soc'y*, 59 Misc.2d 362, 299 N.Y.S.2d 551 (1969). The code of ethics provided that it shall be unethical for any member of the dental society to publish or broadcast any manuscripts or talks to the public dealing with scientific dental matters without first obtaining the society's approval for such broadcast or publications. The constitution and bylaws of the society authorized the suspension or expulsion of any member found guilty of violating the code.

48. The court said that expulsion from membership in the defendants' society would deprive plaintiff

of access to hospital facilities, eligibility for teaching positions, and loss of rights to attend scientific meetings and postgraduate courses sponsored by defendants' society, and reduced malpractice insurance premiums.

49. *Higgins v. Am. Soc'y of Clinical Pathologists*, 51 N.J. 191, 238 A.2d 665 (1968).

50. 51 N.J. 191, 238 A.2d at 669.

51. *Eastern States Retail Lumber Dealers' Ass'n v. United States*, 234 U.S. 600, 34 S.Ct. 951, 953 (1914).

52. In *Fashion Originator's Guild of Am. v. Federal Trade Commission, supra*, note 44, an organization of designers, manufacturers, sellers, and distributors of women's garments and textiles boycotted retailers who sold garments copied from the designs of members of the organization and defended their boycott on the ground that, although not illegal, such sales were unfair trade practices and "tortious invasion[s] of their rights." 312 U.S. at 461, 61 S.Ct. at 705. The court held that, "even if copying were an acknowledged tort under the law of every state, that situation would not justify petitioners in combining together to regulate and restrain interstate commerce in violation of federal law." *Id.* at 468, 61 S.Ct. at 708. *But compare, American Brands, Inc. v. Nat'l Ass'n of Broadcasters*, 308 F.Supp. 1166, 1169–70 (D.D.C. 1969) (held, regulation by a trade association of broadcasters of the content of cigarette advertising carried by members of the association was reasonable as the self-regulation served the public interest.)

53. 317 U.S. 519, 63 S.Ct. 326 (1943).

54. 343 U.S. 326, 72 S.Ct. 690 (1952).

55. *Group Health Coop. v. King County Medical Soc'y*, 39 Wash.2d 586, 237 P.2d 737 (1951).

56. No. C76–168–Y (N.D. Ohio).

57. *In re Medical Serv. Corp. of Spokane County and Medical Serv. Bureau of Spokane County*, 88 FTC 906 (1976).

58. *See, e.g., United States v. Halifax Hosp. Medical Center*, Civ. No. 78–554 (M.D. Fla.) 4 Trade Reg. Rep. (CCH) ¶ 45, 078.

59. *Ohio ex rel Brown v. Alliance Dental Soc'y*, 1976—1 Trade Cases (CCH) ¶ 60,944 (Ohio C.P. 1976).

60. *DeGregorio v. Segal*, 443 F. Supp. 1257 (E.D. Pa. 1978).

61. *Kusick v. San Francisco Council of Nursing Homes*, No. C75–12875W (N.D. Cal. 1975). The Legal Services for the Elderly Poor program in New York City succeeded in ending a threatened boycott by advising the nursing homes involved of the antitrust implications of their actions. *See* Weller, "Medicaid Boycotts and Other Maladies from Medical Monopolists: An Introduction to Antitrust Litigation and the Health Care Industry." 11 *Clearinghouse Rev.* 99, 102–104 (1977).

62. *New York v. Empire City Pharmaceutical Soc'y, Inc.*, 40789/78, N.Y. Sup.Ct. (N.Y. Cty. 1978).

63. *See*, Cheifetz, "The Antitrust Implications of Physician Walkouts," *The Hospital Medical Staff*, June 1976, at 27–30.

64. *Council for Employment and Economic Energy Use v. WHDH Corp.*, 1978—1 Trade Cases (CCH) ¶ 62,101 (1st Cir. 1978); *State of Mo. v. N.O.W., Inc.*, 1979–1 Trade Cases (CCH) ¶ 62507 (W.P. Mo. 1979).

65. *In re Indiana Fed'n of Dentists*, Dkt. No. 9118, FTC, 11–15–78; *In re Indiana Dental Ass'n* File No. 781 0023, F.T.C., 4 Trade Reg. Rptr. ¶ 21,489 (11–18–78).

66. *Feminist Women's Health Center, Inc. v. Mohammad*, 415 F.Supp. 1258 (N.D. Fla. 1976).

67. The local medical society did adopt a resolution to give its moral and financial support to defendants.

68. *Feminist Women's Health Center, Inc. v. Mohammad*, 586 F.2d 530 (5th Cir. 1978).

69. While noting the benefits of product standardization, the FTC has stated that "standards development and certification activities have frequently caused or contributed to substantial consumer and competitive injuries. The injuries include, among others, denial to consumers of the benefits of superior or lower cost technology[,] denial to businesses of the opportunity to enter and compete in profitable industries, inadequate product safety levels, unnecessary costs, and failure to provide for disclosure of important product hazard or use information." FTC, Notice of Proposed Rulemaking, 43 Fed. Reg. 57269, (Dec. 7, 1978) (Supplementary Information).

70. *See Roofire Alarm Co. v. Royal Indemnity Co.*, 202 F.Supp. 166, 169 (E.D. Tenn. 1962). The FTC has stated that "[s]tandards and certifications are relied on extensively in commerce to facilitate communication between sellers and buyers, promote the interchangeability of products and components, transfer technology, assure the safety, fitness and energy efficiency of products, and help achieve efficiencies in design, production and inventory." FTC, Notice of Proposed Rulemaking, 43 Fed. Reg. 57269, (Dec. 7, 1978) (Supplementary Information).

71. *See, e.g., Radio Corp. of Am. v. United States*, 341 U.S. 412, 71 S.Ct. 806 (1951).

72. *See, e.g., Structural Laminates, Inc. v. Douglas Fir Plywood Ass'n*, 261 F. Supp. 154, 156–57 (D. Ore. 1966) (defendant association of plywood manufacturers "played a dominant role in the adoption of Commercial Standards [of the Department of Commerce] for plywood.").

73. *Id.*

74. *Radiant Burners, Inc. v. People's Gas Light and Coke*, 364 U.S. 656, 81 S.Ct. 365 (1961).

75. *Id.; but see, Structural Laminates, Inc. v. Douglas Fir Plywood Ass'n, supra*, note 72, (despite trade association's limiting its seal of approval to members who met its quality standards, conduct of association in evaluating a nonmember's process was reasonable).

76. *United States v. The Am. Soc'y of Mechanical Eng'rs, Inc.*, 1972 Trade Cases (CCH) ¶ 74,028 (S.D. N.Y. 1972) (consent decree).

77. *Tropic Film Corp. v. Paramount Pictures Corp., supra*, note 5 (voluntary program for rating motion pictures held reasonable).

78. FTC, Notice of Proposed Rulemaking, 43 Fed. Reg. 57269, (Dec. 7, 1978) (Summary). The new rule would be at 16 CFR Part 457.

79. *Id.*, at 27270 (Supplementary Information).

80. *Id.*, at 27269 (Supplementary Information).

81. *See*, pages 133–136.

82. *Milk and Ice Cream Can Inst. v. Federal Trade Commission*, 152 F.2d 478, 482 (7th Cir. 1946).

83. 345 F.2d 421 (7th Cir. 1965).

84. See section on certification, *supra*.

85. *United States v. Socony-Vacuum Oil Co.*, 310 U.S. 150, 60 S.Ct. 811, 842–43 (1940).

86. *Id.*, at 221, 60 S.Ct. at 843. ("The reasonableness of prices has no constancy due to the dynamic quality of the business facts underlying price structures. Those who fixed reasonable prices today would perpetuate unreasonable prices tomorrow, since those prices would not be subject to continuous administrative supervision and readjustment in light of changed conditions. . . . Any combination which tampers with price structures is engaged in an unlawful activity. Even though the members of the price-fixing group were in no position to control the market, to the extent that they raised, lowered, or stabilized prices they would be directly interfering with the free play of market forces.")

87. *See, e.g., United States v. Nat'l Ass'n of Real Estate Bds.*, 339 U.S. 485, 70 S.Ct. 711 (1950); *United States v. Rental Nationwide Trailer Rental Sys., Inc.*, 156 F.Supp. 800 (D. Kan. 1957) (price fixing held unlawful despite fact that defendant was essentially a joint venture, but where membership was restricted by geographic area.)

88. *Plymouth Dealers' Ass'n of N. California v. United States*, 279 F.2d 128, 132–33 (9th Cir. 1960). The court also emphasized that even if ineffective, an agreement to fix prices would by itself be unlawful. *See also, United States v. Nat'l Ass'n of Real Estate Bds.*, *supra* note 87, 339 U.S. at 489, 70 S.Ct. at 714. (An agreement to fix prices is unlawful even without provision for enforcement; "the fact that no penalties are imposed for deviations from the price schedules is not material.") *See also, Federal Trade Commission v. Pacific States Paper Trade Ass'n*, 273 U.S. 52, 47 S.Ct. 255 (1927).

89. *See, e.g., United States v. American Soc'y of Civil Eng'rs*, 446 F. Supp. 803 (S.D. N.Y. 1977).

90. *See, e.g., United States v. Nat'l Ass'n of Real Estate Bds.*, *supra*, note 88, 339 U.S. 489–92, 70 S.Ct. 714–16.

91. *Supra*, note 14.

92. In *Goldfarb* the issue was whether the Virginia State Bar could enforce a fee schedule published by a local bar association that included minimum prices for title examinations, a service that only a lawyer could perform and that was a prerequisite for the purchase of a house. Every lawyer plaintiff homebuyers contacted adhered to the published fee schedule, which was enforced by the state bar. The court found that "in terms of restraining competition and harming consumers . . . the price-fixing activities found here are unusually damaging. A title examination is indispensable in the process of financing a real estate purchase, and since only an attorney licensed to practice in Virginia may legally examine a title . . . consumers could not turn to alternative sources for the necessary service." 421 U.S. 782, 95 S.Ct. 2010 (1975).

93. 421 U.S. 788, n.17, 95 S.Ct. 2013, n.17 (1975).

94. *National Soc'y of Professional Eng'rs v. United States*, U.S., 98 S.Ct. 1355 (1978).

95. *Id.*, at 98 S.Ct. 1367.

96. *See, e.g., Massachusetts v. Massachusetts Nurses Ass'n*, No. 31921 (Mass. Super., Suffolk County, November 14, 1978) (an association of nurses who contracted independently to give nursing care to individual patients allegedly fixed prices in violation of state antitrust act by promulgating uniform rate schedules for private duty nursing care intended to serve as minimum fees.)

97. Trade Reg. Rep. (CCH) ¶ 21,475 (Oct. 16, 1978).

98. *Bates v. State Bar of Arizona*, 97 S.Ct. 2691 (1977).

99. *American Brands, Inc. v. Nat'l Ass'n of Broadcasters*, 308 F. Supp. 1166 (D.D.C. 1969).

100. *The American Medical Ass'n*, Trade Reg. Rep. (CCH) ¶ 21,491, 21,525 (1978).

101. National Health Council Government Relations Note, Antitrust and Health Services: A Second Look, A Special Report Including a Chronology of Antitrust Actions 1975–1978 (June 1978).

102. *Id.*

103. 451 F. Supp. 624 (W.D. Va. 1978).

104. In *Bartholomew* plaintiffs were chiropractors with theories of chiropractic different from those of members of the defendant association. They contended that under their theories the amount of treatment they gave their patients at each office was much more than that given by association chiropractors, and therefore that the association's maximum fee for an office visit was below the fair fee for plaintiff's services. Consequently, they contended that adherence to the fee resulted in a boycott of plaintiffs, since they could not have the entire fee reimbursed.

105. The court was considering defendants' motions for judgment on the pleadings, dismissal, and the quashing of process.

106. *See also, Blue Cross of Virginia v. Commonwealth of Virginia*, 1970 Trade Cases (CCH) ¶ 73,316 (Va. 1970), where the principal agreement was between a health care insurer, Blue Cross, and pharmacists, under which the pharmacists agreed to furnish prescription drugs to Blue Cross subscribers at a price equal to cost plus a professional fee of $1.85 per prescription. The court found

that the State Pharmaceutical Association, although not a defendant, had facilitated an agreement among all the pharmacists to set the prices of all prescriptions according to the Blue Cross formula. While each contract was with a separate pharmacist, the court found, in part on the basis of promotion of Blue Cross appearances before the association, that "[n]one of the pharmacists who contracted with Blue Cross for the supplying of drugs could have reasonably believed that his contract was an isolated transaction. Each must have known that Blue Cross entered into the contract pursuant to a plan that required for success the making of the same contract with other pharmacists across the State." 1970 Trade Cases at p. 89,248.

107. *The American College of Radiology*, Order, Dkt. C–2871, March 1, 1977, Trade Reg. Rep. (CCH) ¶ 21,236.

108. 334 U.S. 219, 68 S.Ct. 996 (1948).

109. "It is clear that the agreement is the sort of combination condemned by the [Sherman] Act, even though the price-fixing was by purchasers, and the persons specially injured under the treble damage claim are sellers, not customers or consumers." *Id.*, at 235, 68 S.Ct. 1005–06.

110. *See*, discussion of conspiracy in Chapter 1.

111. *United States v. Consolidated Packaging Corp.*, 575 F.2d 117, 127 (7th Cir. 1978) ("We deem it irrelevant that Consolidated did not know all the other conspirators, or have knowledge of all the transactions in which it had no immediate interest. It is well understood that a conspirator need not know all the other conspirators, nor have direct contact with them.")

112. *American Tobacco Co. v. United States*, 328 U.S. 781, 809, 66 S.Ct. 1125, 1139 (1946) ("It is not the form of the combination or the particular means used but the result to be achieved that the statute condemns. It is not of importance whether the means used to accomplish the unlawful objective are in themselves lawful or unlawful. Acts done to give effect to the conspiracy may be in themselves wholly innocent acts.")

113. *United States v. Am. Linseed Oil Co.*, 262 U.S. 371, 43 S.Ct. 607 (1923); *see also, Sugar Inst. v. United States*, 297 U.S. 553, 601, 56 S.Ct. 629, 643 (1936) ("The unreasonable restraint which defendants imposed lay not in advance announcements, but in the steps taken to secure adherence, without deviation, to prices and terms thus announced.")

114. *Tag Mfrs. Inst. v. Federal Trade Commission*, 174 F.2d 452 (1st Cir. 1949).

115. *American Column & Lumber Co. v. United States*, 257 U.S. 377 412, 42 S.Ct. 114, 121 (1921) (dissenting).

116. *United States v. Am. Linseed Oil Co., supra*, note 113, 262 U.S. 390, 43 S.Ct. 611–12 (1923). *See also, Sugar Inst. v. United States, supra*, note 113, 297 U.S. 598–99, 56 S.Ct. 642 (1936).

117. *Sugar Inst. v. United States*, 297 U.S. 553, 56 S.Ct. 629 (1936).

118. *Id.*, at 597, 56 S.Ct. 641.

119. *See, e.g., Maple Flooring Mfrs. Ass'n v. United States*, 268 U.S. 563, 45 S.Ct. 578 (1925); *Tag Mfrs. Inst. v. Federal Trade Commission, supra*, note *114*.

120. *American Column & Lumber Co. v. United States, supra*, note 115, 257 U.S. 398, 42 S.Ct. 116.

121. Thus, in *Tag Mfrs. Inst. v. Federal Trade Commission, supra*, note 114, where the products of the members of the association rarely were standardized, the court found that distribution of price lists did not have the effect of restricting price competition. *Compare, Sugar Inst. v. United States, supra*, note 113, where the product, sugar, was totally standardized and price was the only means of competition. *See also, United States Maltsters Ass'n v. Federal Trade Commission*, 152 F.2d 161, 166 (7th Cir. 1945).

122. *Sugar Inst. v. United States, supra*, note 113.

123. *Belliston v. Texaco, Inc.*, 455 F.2d 175 (10th Cir. 1972).

124. *See, supra*, pp. 132–133.

125. Trade Reg. Rep. (CCH) ¶ 50,340.

126. *Id.*, at 55,719–20.

127. 393 U.S. 333, 89 S.Ct. 510 (1969).

128. *Id.*, at 336, 89 S.Ct. 512. In *Container Corp.*, the communication of price information was by way of an informal agreement under which executives of competing sellers of corrugated containers would ask each other for recent price information, with formal procedures for sharing such information and without an agreement to adhere to the prices received. However, there was an expectation that one who gave price information to another would, in turn, be given price information if he asked for it.

129. *Id.*, at 338, 89 S.Ct. 513.

130. *Id.*, at 338–39, 89 S.Ct. 513 (Fortas, J., concurring). "There is no single test to determine when the record adequately shows an 'unreasonable restraint of trade'; but a practice such as that here involved, which is adopted for the purpose of arriving at a determination of prices to be quoted to individual customers, inevitably suggests the probability that it so materially interfered with the operation of the price mechanism of the market place as to bring it within the condemnation of this Court's decisions."

131. *United States v. Citizens and Southern Nat'l Bank*, 422 U.S. 86, 113, 95 S.Ct. 2099, 2115 (1975); *see also, Belliston v. Texaco, Inc., supra*, note 123, 455 F.2d at 181.

132. *Supra*, note 115.

133. *Supra*, note 113.

134. *Supra*, note 113.

135. *Cement Mfrs. Protective Ass'n v. United States*, 268 U.S. 588, 604, 45 S.Ct. 586, 591 (1925); *United States v. Fur Dressers' and Fur Dyers' Ass'n*, 5 F.2d 869 (S.D. N.Y. 1925); *United States v. S. California Wholesale Grocers' Ass'n*, 7 F.2d 944 (S.D. Cal. 1925); *Michelman v. Clark-Schwebel Fiberglass Corp.*, 534 F.2d 1036, 1048 (2nd Cir. 1976) (held, exchanging credit information permissible, so long as no agreement to act on it). *But see, Swift and Co. v. United States*, 196 U.S. 375, 25 S.Ct. 276 (1905) (one aspect of an enjoined conspiracy in restraint of trade was defendants' attempt to set a uniform rule for granting credit to customers.) As an associational benefit, access to credit facilities may not generally be restricted to members. *United States v. Allied Florists Ass'n of Ill.*, 1953 Trade Cases (CCH) ¶ 67,433 (M.D. Ill. 1953) (consent decree).

136. 15 U.S.C. § 13(a) *et seq.*

137. *Standard Motor Parts v. Federal Trade Commission*, 265 F.2d 674, 676–77 (2d Cir. 1959); *see also, Am. Motor Specialties Co. v. Federal Trade Commission*, 278 F.2d 225 (2d Cir. 1960).

138. *Standard Motor Products, Inc. v. Federal Trade Commission, supra*, note *137*, 265 F.2d 677; *Federal Trade Commission v. Cement Inst.*, 333 U.S 683, 721–26, 68 S.Ct. 793, 813–16 (1948).

139. *See, e.g., Standard Motor Products, Inc. v. Federal Trade Commission, supra*, note 137; *Am. Motor Specialties Co. v. Federal Trade Commission, supra*, note 137.

140. *Alhambra Motor Parts v. Federal Trade Commission*, 309 F.2d 213, 217–21 (9th Cir. 1962); *but compare, Gen. Auto Supplies, Inc. v. Federal Trade Commission*, 346 F.2d 311 (1965) (despite the fact that cooperative buyer warehoused products for its members, held, it still did not itself sell to the members, and therefore price discounts were in violation of the Robinson-Patman Act.).

141. 405 U.S. 596, 92 S.Ct. 1126 (1972).

142. 405 U.S. 605–09, 92 S.Ct. 1132–34.

143. *See, supra*, pp. 109–111. [re: membership - reasonable exclusions].

144. *Cf., American Fed'n of Tobacco Growers, Inc. v. Neal, supra*, note 4.

145. 365 U.S. 127, 81 S.Ct. 523 (1961).

146. "It is neither unusual nor illegal for people to seek action on laws in the hope that they may bring about an advantage to themselves and a disadvantage to their competitors." 365 U.S. at 139, 81 S.Ct. at 530. The Court reiterated this doctrine in *United Mine Workers of America v. Pennington*, 381 U.S. 657, 85 S.Ct. 1585 (1965).

147. 365 U.S. 144, 81 S.Ct. 533 (1961).

148. 404 U.S. 508, 92 S.Ct. 609 (1972).

149. *Id.*, at 512, 92 S.Ct. 612.

Chapter 6

Medical Staff Privileges and Related Issues

The continuing business relations between hospitals and physicians inevitably lead to legal disputes of various natures. Issues that frequently involve restraint of trade, and therefore are within the scope of this chapter, generally relate to questions of whether, or under what conditions, physicians will enjoy staff privileges at a particular facility. In essence, the single most important issue in this area is the right of a hospital to refuse to deal, or to restrict the conditions upon which it will deal, with physicians.

The question of the right to medical staff privileges generally arises in one of two broad categories: (1) closed staff denials of privileges, where physicians are denied privileges for reasons unrelated to the individual physician, as where a hospital determines to operate a department under an exclusive departmental contract; and (2) open staff denials, where a particular physician is denied privileges for reasons peculiar to that individual. Each of these circumstances raises potentially distinct issues and consequently must be analyzed separately by the facility, as well as in this chapter.

THE CLOSED STAFF

Competitive restrictions emanating from the closure of medical staffs, primarily relating to exclusive departmental arrangements, are among the more frequently litigated restraint-of-trade issues in the health care industry. The reasons for this frequency are not difficult to discern. Few, if any, hospitals have avoided the temptation to simplify and perhaps stabilize and economize the operation of particular departments through exclusive contracts. These arrangements can offer the hospital dependability in hours and methods of operating specialized departments, among other benefits.

The decision to go exclusive, however, is not without its negative implications. An exclusive arrangement with a physician or a group of physicians means that others, perhaps equally talented and skillful, are precluded from this professional opportunity. In some instances, the department that is closed to others than the fortunate contracting physician may be the only one of its kind in the vicinity. Consequently, physicians desiring to pursue the now-precluded specialty either must work for the contracting physician, leave the area, or challenge the exclusive arrangement.

The courts' analysis of the validity of the exclusive departmental contracts, while occasionally involving quite different legal bases, have followed remarkably consistent approaches. Of primary importance throughout the courts' analyses are certain basic rules of self-protection, repeatedly cited for the benefit of all parties. Specifically, the cases demonstrate the value of following proper administrative procedures before going exclusive in a department. As with any antitrust analysis, the rules and guidelines discussed by the courts must form the basis for predicting and, it is hoped, avoiding trouble areas, as the statutory framework is too broad to be of substantial practical value.

Consequently, this chapter first considers representative closed staff cases listed in published court opinions. Because of the rapid changes in the law subsequent to many of these cases and the apparent trend toward standardizing the approach taken in antitrust cases in the health care industry with those in other industries, the chapter then evaluates potential changes and sensitive areas through analogy to cases involving other industries.

Traditional Closed Staff Cases

Most of the reported court decisions on exclusive departmental contracts were reached in an era when the medical profession, as other professions, was considered exempt from the antitrust laws because of the then-perceived "learned professions" concept and the belief that the practice of medicine was not part of, and did not affect, interstate commerce in a way that invoked federal jurisdiction. There have been occasional analytical shifts among the cases, some relying solely on theories of common law tort, others on state and even federal antitrust principles, and still others on constitutional principles. However, the factors on which the courts have based the validity of exclusive arrangements, and the guidelines to be gleaned from the analyses, are quite similar.

Perhaps the best known of the cases analyzing exclusive departmental agreements for antitrust type violations is the 1965 California decision known as *Blank v. Palo Alto-Stanford Hospital Center*.[1] The hospital in this case had contracted with a physician group, giving it the exclusive right to operate the hospital's radiology department. The group, in turn, subcontracted with a physician partnership for some of the physician services. The plaintiff, a Dr. Blank, had been a member of the radiology department staff before the contract and was excluded from that staff when the deal was signed. Dr. Blank charged that the contract violated the Cartwright Act, California's state antitrust law (which substantially parallels federal antitrust law).

During the trial of the *Blank* case, the California Supreme Court handed down its decision in *Willis v. Santa Ana Hospital Association*,[2] holding in part that the medical profession was exempt from the Cartwright Act,[3] and explaining that in refusal to deal situations, common law created a cause of action where the right to pursue a lawful calling or occupation was interfered with intentionally, either by unlawful means or by lawful means but without justification.

The court in *Blank* pursued this common law theory of interference with the pursuit of a lawful trade, declaring that an exclusive dealing arrangement such as this could not be, in and of itself, a violation of any known law. As the hospital had pursued a somewhat formal administrative procedure before deciding to go exclusive, the court ruled that it would not reverse this administrative decision unless the decision was found to violate recognized rights, such as the right to pursue a lawful trade or calling. The court said the question of good medical practice, as determined by the hospital, was purely administrative in nature, involving no legal principle.

The court decided radiology was a medical service and not merely a hospital service (perhaps casting doubt on the applicability of this analysis to such hospital services as dietary and laundry). The court determined that a violation of the law would be established only if: (1) there was interference with the plaintiff's right to practice his calling and, either, (2) that interference was by unlawful means or (3) was by means otherwise lawful but without justification in this instance.

The court appeared to have little difficulty finding that the exclusive dealing contract, as a practical matter, inhibited the plaintiff's ability to practice medicine to the full extent he desired. It then analyzed arguments of justification, applying the general standards of considering: (1) the appropriateness of the conduct as a means of advancing legitimate interests, and (2) the availability of less harmful means to the same end. The court specifically noted that the unreasonableness of a contract that restrains trade depends not only on the resulting monopoly but on whether the purpose of the contract is the creation of the monopoly and whether that monopoly enjoys a dominant social or economic justification.

The court found the exclusive contract justified for the following reasons:

- The hospital had conducted an extensive study of ways of furnishing legally required radiology services. It had discussed possibilities at several board meetings and had determined that it could best discharge its legal duty through an exclusive dealing contract with radiologists selected by the board.
- The board specifically found that outpatient care would be improved and

hospital administration efficiency increased because the exclusive contract would:

1. facilitate the administration and supervision of the department and improve interrelationships between the department and the rest of the hospital
2. assure immediate availability of specialized physicians and assure requisite coverage at odd hours
3. simplify scheduling among otherwise competing radiologists, thus allowing patient needs to take precedence over factors of competition
4. provide continuous consultation availability
5. emulate similar contracts then used by substantially all hospitals in the country

The court further determined that the exclusive arrangement caused no material damage to the public, financial or otherwise, and found this to be a reasonable rule or regulation that the governing board of the hospital was entitled to adopt.

The *Blank* decision has been relied upon in subsequent exclusive contract cases in California and other states. For example, the general rules of *Blank* were applied specifically to a publicly owned and operated hospital in *Letsch v. Northern San Diego County Hospital District*.[4] In that 1966 case, the California Supreme Court ruled that the situation was identical to *Blank* except that the hospital was operated by a public agency. The court held that this fact made no difference to the legality of the exclusive departmental arrangement. As in *Blank*, the hospital in *Letsch* had pursued an administrative proceeding before deciding to go exclusive.

The *Blank* decision was followed in a third California case, in *Lewin v. St. Joseph Hospital of Orange*[5] in 1978. Unlike *Blank* and *Letsch*, the *Lewin* case involved a hospital's decision to go exclusive in its chronic hemodialysis service. The hospital also had followed an extensive administrative procedure before signing the exclusive agreement and, as in the previous cases, this weighed heavily in the court's decision. During the administrative process, the aggrieved physician was given the opportunity to present his views to the executive committee of the hospital medical staff. The executive committee also analyzed the relative merits of operating the hemodialysis unit on a closed staff, as compared to an open staff, basis. In its decision, the court offered one statement of general applicability in all similar cases. In explaining its review of the hospital's decision to go exclusive, the court enunciated the general principle that:

A managerial decision concerning operation of the hospital made rationally and in good faith by the Board to which operation of the hospital is committed by law should not be countermanded by the courts unless it clearly appears it is unlawful or will seriously injure a significant public interest.[6]

The court also analyzed the conduct of the hospital under rules applicable to association activities, relying on the general principle that: "Whenever a private association is legally required to refrain from arbitrary action, the association's action must be substantively rational and procedurally fair."[7] In determining that the hospital's decision to go exclusive was not arbitrary or capricious, the court in *Lewin* also coincided with the *Blank* standards in relying on the fact that the majority of hospitals in the area apparently operated their chronic hemodialysis units on a closed staff basis. In sum, the court in *Lewin* extended tremendous deference to the administrative decision of the hospital and held that closure of the chronic hemodialysis unit did not constitute an unreasonable restraint of trade nor an unreasonable interference with the physician's right to pursue his trade or calling.[8]

A 1975 decision of the Arizona Court of Appeals in *Dattilo v. Tucson General Hospital*,[9] in approving the legality of an exclusive departmental contract, offered the perhaps simplifying virtue of explaining that the applicable analysis under the common law tort of unreasonable interference with a trade or calling was identical to that of the Arizona state antitrust law, and that that law could be analyzed under standards applicable to the Sherman Act. The Arizona court then applied the test established in cases under the Sherman Act to both the common law and the state antitrust law. It also relied upon *Blank* and similar analyses. The plaintiff in *Dattilo* was an osteopath, and the geographic area in which he practiced supported only one osteopathic hospital. Consequently, the practice of his profession, to the extent that he relied upon hospital services, could be pursued only at the defendant hospital.

This hospital, in its effort to attract more certified internists to its staff, agreed to give a particular physician it desired a five-year exclusive contract to operate the hospital's nuclear medicine service. The plaintiff, who was not a board-certified internist, meanwhile had been studying nuclear medicine and had received a license to practice in this specialty from the Arizona Atomic Energy Commission. In fact, he had begun practicing this service at the defendant hospital before the exclusive nuclear department service contract was signed. The plaintiff proposed that the hospital grant him privileges to conduct the nuclear medicine department. When the hospital rejected this proposal in favor of the exclusive contract with the newly attracted board-certified internist, the plaintiff sued under the Arizona state antitrust law and common law, charging unreasonable restraint of trade.

The plaintiff in *Dattilo* sought to distinguish his situation from previous cases because in this instance the defendant hospital was the only one in which he could practice in his immediate geographical area. The court, however, ruled that the situation was similar to that in *Blank, Letsch*, and other cases because, even though the plaintiff was precluded from practicing nuclear medicine, he did retain his general staff privileges in internal medicine, so he was not entirely precluded from practicing his profession.

On the question of reasonableness and justification of the exclusive arrangement, the court held that:

1. The exclusive contract was necessary to control and standardize procedures and the operation of the nuclear medicine department;
2. The exclusive contract gave the hospital's board of trustees the ability to ensure quality standards by monitoring the department, since fewer persons would participate there;
3. Patient care would be improved because of better scheduling and higher quality results;
4. The service would operate economically;
5. The exclusive contract assured the consistency of technicians' training;
6. The contract would allow doctors to keep up with current cases in the field;
7. The contract would create a pool of medical knowledge available to all staff members.

The court also relied on the universality of this type of arrangement in nuclear medicine departments. Thus, while the Arizona court appeared to recognize the general applicability of standards developed under the antitrust statutes, the actual analysis and result were virtually identical to the *Blank* decision, which was reached entirely under the common law tort theory.

The relatively early (1950) case of *Jeanes v. Burke*[10] focused on the consideration of the length of time during which the exclusive contract was to operate. In this case, a Texas hospital entered into an exclusive contract with a single physician, granting that individual the exclusive right to conduct major surgery in the hospital for five years. Although the court found the contract not to be void for creating a monopoly, its analysis was quite different from that of later decisions. In particular, the court relied upon the fact that the institution was not owned by the general public and was not operated by the governing body of a city or county. It also appeared to assume other antitrust standards did not apply. Where ordinary exclusive dealing standards are applied, however, it is appropriate to consider the length of the contractual term, with a preference for shorter terms where practical.

One of the few federal decisions analyzing staff privileges is found in *Harron v. United Hospital Center, Inc.*[11] The 1975 *Harron* case presents the anomaly of a physician who previously had been granted an exclusive departmental contract suing, in part, on an antitrust theory when he lost that contract after two hospitals merged. During the period when the two hospitals coexisted in the vicinity of the plaintiff's practice, Harron had been the exclusive radiologist at one hospital and another physician was the exclusive radiologist at the other. When the hospitals merged, they temporarily operated an open staff radiology department. The open staff radiology department proved unsatisfactory, and the surviving hospital granted an exclusive contract to a physician other than the plaintiff. Harron sued, contending that the exclusive contract violated both the Sherman Act and his civil rights. The court concluded, however, that such a contention was frivolous and dismissed the action. This federal court, unlike previous state courts analyzing similar circumstances, did not even offer a detailed analysis of the justifications for such an exclusive arrangement.

Variations on the Exclusive Contract Theme

A number of other cases, most of them slight variations on the exclusive contract theme, demonstrate that the general standards and analyses described apply to virtually any situation dealing with the impact of a staff closure, whether the closure is as explicit and well-defined as an exclusive contract or is created by more subtle or intricate means.

In *Benell v. City of Virginia*,[12] a public hospital had adopted a resolution requiring that all x-rays there be taken under the supervision of the single hospital radiologist. The plaintiff physician sued, based upon this resolution, contending that it was not satisfactory for a radiologist, such as the plaintiff, to be required to look at films taken by another radiologist. Although this 1960 Minnesota case was not brought under antitrust statutes and the common law tort cited in *Blank* was not identified specifically, the court's analysis was quite similar to that in *Blank* and other later cases. In particular, the court said its only function was to analyze whether the hospital commission's action in adopting the resolution was arbitrary or unreasonable. It added that it would not attempt to determine whether the hospital's action was a better course of conduct than that requested by the plaintiff. Based on evidence on the propriety of the resolution, the court held that the resolution was reasonable and valid.[13]

A slight variation on the exclusive departmental contract theme is found in the 1967 Florida case of *Rush v. City of Saint Petersburg*.[14] In this situation, the defendant city owned and operated a hospital and entered into a contract with a single radiologist providing that all "unassigned" radiological cases would be handled by this individual. The plaintiff, a competing radiologist, sued to enjoin the city and the contracting physician on the theory that the contract constituted the illegal corporate practice of medicine by the municipal hospital. Consequently, the case was not determined on antitrust grounds, and the court did not explore the common law theories followed in *Blank*. However, the court did specifically evaluate whether the performance of the contract adversely affected the public welfare, and determined that it did not.

As in *Rush*, the decision in *Adler v. Montefiore Hospital Association of Western Pennsylvania*[15] was not reached on antitrust principles. However, the court in *Adler*, under constitutional standards, did analyze hospital regulations that permitted only the full-time director of the hospital's laboratory to perform cardiac catheterizations and related procedures. In so doing, the court demonstrated once again the similarity of the appropriate analysis of these types of exclusive departmental arrangements, no matter what law was said to apply. In particular, it received expert testimony on the impact of the exclusive arrangement and concluded that the practice improved patient care, the hospital's teaching program, and the efficient administration of the hospital for the following reasons:

1. The procedures performed were essentially team functions, and the exclusive arrangement allowed the members of the team to develop a routine and familiarity with the equipment and its use by a particular physician;
2. The exclusive operator's full-time presence at the hospital allowed that individual to treat complications with patients upon whom he performed procedures;
3. If more than one physician performed the procedures, there would not be enough of them to assure continued competence because the hospital had relatively few of these cases;
4. The arrangement allowed the exclusive operator to teach students, interns, and residents effectively;
5. The arrangement relieved scheduling problems that otherwise would be created by staff members who had outside commitments;
6. The arrangement apparently improved the ability of the physician to schedule procedures in the morning so that complications could be treated in the afternoon;
7. The arrangement improved the ability of the exclusive operator to handle important administrative details;
8. The arrangement reduced the probability of equipment breakdowns;
9. As the hospital could be liable for malpractice injuries, it had a legitimate interest in ensuring the optimal performance of its employees and of its equipment.

Notably, although the analysis in *Adler* proceeded along constitutional lines and although the hospital did not rely explicitly upon an internal administrative proceeding in reaching the decision to go exclusive, the factors relied upon by the court should emphasize again the importance of creating a proper administrative record to establish the public value of this type of decision through a demonstration of an improvement in the quality of medical care.

A somewhat different, and in some ways less defensible, closed staff situation was *Guerrero v. Burlington County Memorial Hospital*.[16] In fact, the 1976

Guerrero case presents the issue of the totally closed surgical staff, as opposed to the closed department. The *Guerrero* case involved, first, the establishment of a "satellite hospital" (a creature of New Jersey Law), designed primarily to provide a facility for the treatment of urgent and emergency cases in a particular community region. After the satellite facility had been established, it proved so successful that surgical and occupancy statistics demonstrated to the satisfaction of the medical executive committee that any further growth in surgical services would be likely to result in a reduction of the quality of care. Consequently, the hospital determined after an administrative proceeding not to allow any further expansion of the surgical staff.

Two new surgeons in the area thus were denied privileges at the hospital and sued to have the staff closure decision reversed. The court did not refer to any antitrust statutes, relying entirely upon general rules of law applicable to the operation of hospitals in that state. The analysis, however, recognized and applied a deference to the decisions of the hospital administration identical to that in exclusive departmental cases from other states. The court noted the importance to surgeons of having staff privileges, since they otherwise would be unable to pursue their professions. Of counterbalancing importance, however, was the interest in maintaining the quality of patient care. The court decided not to perform an actual balancing test itself, but confined its analysis to determining whether the hospital's decision was supported by substantial, credible evidence and was neither arbitrary nor capricious.

The court held that the decision of the hospital administration to close the staff was not arbitrary or capricious and was supported by substantial evidence introduced during the hospital's own administrative decision-making process. The court explained, however, that the hospital's right to deny staff privileges could not be extended to routine denials motivated by a simple desire to exclude newcomers in order to protect the position of existing staff members. Thus, even where the decision to close a hospital staff is not related to a medical necessity of granting exclusive privileges to conduct specialized procedures, but is based simply on the overcrowding of the hospital facility, the analysis in at least this instance is essentially the same.

A New Jersey state court in 1969 addressed a similar issue, where a hospital restricted the staff of its obstetrics-gynecology department because of excessively high occupancy. The court explicitly applied the standards in *Blank*, encouraged hospital boards to create proper records demonstrating how they reached such decisions, and ruled that the hospital had acted reasonably in these circumstances.[17] The court cautioned, however, that when occupancy became more manageable, the staff restrictions would not be acceptable.

Seven years later, however, another New Jersey state court considered a challenge to a hospital staff moratorium that again had been motivated by excessively high occupancy rates, and found this staff closure to violate constitutional standards.[18] The court particularly noted that occupancy statistics had not changed significantly after the moratorium began and that this hospital historically had enjoyed a census approaching 100 percent. As there was no evidence demonstrating that the moratorium was necessary or even beneficial in protecting the quality of care at the hospital, the court declared there was no justification for the staff closure. Had there been evidence demonstrating a need for the moratorium to assure the quality of care, the court indicated it would have permitted it to continue. In these circumstances, however, it said the closure served merely to preserve the positions of established staff members and to discriminate against new physicians. Although this case was not decided on an antitrust basis, little analysis is required to indicate that a demonstration that the moratorium was the result of a conspiracy between the hospital and various staff members could have resulted in a treble damage award to the excluded physicians. A proper record on protection of the quality of care, however, might have prevented the problem altogether.

Caveats

These cases help demonstrate that, to this point, the courts have extended a general deference to hospital conduct on staff closures. This is especially true where there is some sort of previous administrative proceeding upon which the court may rely. The descriptions of the evidence offered at trial also lead to the conclusion that the plaintiff physicians may have been less than thorough in the presentation of their cases. Furthermore, the cases evaluated under various state laws and various types of legal theories apply an apparently similar analysis of potentially justifying factors for the staff closures, irrespective of which body of law the plaintiffs sought to invoke. In at least one of the more extensively reasoned cases, the court professed a belief that it was attempting to apply a traditional Sherman Act (and similar state antitrust law) rule of reason analysis to a staff closure.

With the demise of the learned professions exemption, which previously may have helped insulate staff closure situations from explicit review under the Sherman Act or similar state antitrust laws,[19] as well as significant changes in traditional doctrines relating to finding the requisite impact upon interstate commerce,[20] and with the increasing importance of exclusive dealing arrangements to the practices of individual physicians, it seems reasonable to expect an increase in the tendency to litigate such cases in Federal court under Sherman Act standards or in state courts under analogous state laws. If, as seems reasonable, it then may be assumed that litigants in actions of this type will more heavily rely upon a professed application of Sherman Act standards, it must be worthwhile to consider how the federal courts apply the Sherman Act to exclusive dealing arrangements in other industries.

In this type of analysis, however, the first problem is that relatively few exclusive dealing cases have been decided under the Sherman Act. This is primarily a result of the availability of Section 3 of the Clayton Act, which is more directly applicable to, and more restrictive of, exclusive dealing contracts. This section applies, however, only to arrangements involving the purchases or sales of commodities, and thus is inapplicable to exclusive service contracts such as the exclusive departmental arrangements considered here.

Of those cases available involving the Sherman Act, a particularly helpful application is offered by the U.S. Court of Appeals for the Third Circuit in the 1975 case of *American Motor Inns, Inc., v. Holiday Inns, Inc.*[21] The *Holiday Inns* case is useful for several reasons. First, the analysis arose in the context of a contractual clause Holiday Inns imposed on its franchisees requiring that they not compete with the franchisor during the term of the franchise agreement. In form, this basic covenant not to compete was a requirement that franchisees of Holiday Inn motels not own motels other than those in the Holiday Inn chain. The court treated this type of in-term (meaning that it is effective only during the contractual relationship) covenant not to compete as an exclusive dealing arrangement under the standard Sherman Act rule of reason, applicable to any other exclusive dealing contract. The case thereby demonstrates that health care facilities that may desire to make their exclusive departmental contracts into two-way streets (meaning that the physician or physicians who obtain the exclusive right to operate the department are reciprocally prohibited from competing with the hospital by practicing elsewhere during the term of the contract) may determine the legality of this type of reciprocal arrangement under the same standards as apply to ordinary, unilateral exclusive contracts.[22]

Second, the court in *Holiday Inns* explained that the rule of reason standard to be applied in Sherman Act exclusive dealing cases was interchangeable with that of other situations, as it expressly relied upon what is generally considered the leading statement of rule of reason analysis, the 1918 case of *Board of Trade of City of Chicago v. United States*.[23]

A detailed consideration of the many ways in which the rule of reason has been applied to other industries, and the individual merits of the elements of justification of the hospital cases mentioned, would be cumbersome. However, it is worthwhile to consider whether state courts that may profess to apply a standard rule of reason analysis in exclusive departmental cases are being entirely candid. This question must be asked particularly with respect to the state courts' repeated reliance on the universality of the exclusive dealing method as an element of justification in and of itself.

In other analyses, the prevalence of exclusive arrangements over otherwise available market outlets has been perceived to be a significant negative factor in determining the legality of the deal, as such a circumstance demonstrates that most market alternatives no longer are available to the now excluded, would-be new entrant (the physician seeking to practice in spite of the exclusive contract). In fact, the anticompetitive evil against which the exclusive dealing rules of law are applied is the foreclosure of competitive outlets for the service or product of a plaintiff. Generally, the more pervasive the market foreclosure, the more likely that the exclusive arrangement will be found illegal.

The justification factors so often repeated in similar fashion by state courts may constitute a significant rationalization supporting demonstrably responsible, quality-oriented hospital conduct, stemming from a perhaps well-founded judicial reluctance to tamper with the quality of medical care in the absence of overwhelming evidence requiring such intervention.

A third point of interest in the *Holiday Inns* case is the fact that an agreement that otherwise would not violate the Sherman Act rule of reason becomes a violation if the agreement was designed to achieve a forbidden restraint, such as where it was intended to be part of a scheme to monopolize, to fix prices, or to drive a competitor out of the market. Consequently, the demonstration of a proper intent in closing a staff becomes extremely important.

It is hoped that all of these considerations will lead facilities desiring to expand the scope of their exclusive operations, or to close staffs for other reasons, to maintain good administrative records, demonstrating the painstaking and open analysis they have made in reaching their decisions. This appears to be at least one very viable method of improving the opportunities for receiving judicial deference to the hospital's decision, as well as perhaps improving the quality of that decision when it is made. Notably, the court in *Holiday Inns* explicitly rejected a contention that an exclusive dealing arrangement must be invalidated if it is not the least restrictive means of reaching the parties' legitimate goals. Rather, it said, restrictive arrangements need only be "fairly necessary" in the circumstances of the particular case. Thus, the parameters within which the hospital's administrative decision-making process will be held valid enjoy some breadth and, while the facility should demonstrate that it has considered other means of achieving the desired goal, it will not become a guarantor that it has chosen the least restrictive means.

These state cases, as well as the general rules on exclusive dealing (discussed briefly in Chapter 1), assume that the hospital that decides to go exclusive is not a direct competitor with the physicians who thus are precluded from offering their services in that now exclusive department. Ordinarily, of course, hospitals and physicians are not competitors in the marketplace in that sense, but rather offer complementary services to patients. Where, however, the hospital that goes exclusive is owned or controlled by the physicians who are the beneficiaries of that arrangement, additional considerations may apply. In that type of circumstance, physicians excluded from practicing at the particular hospital, and perhaps in an entire locality, may attempt to demonstrate that what appears to be an essentially vertical exclusive dealing arrangement is in fact a horizontal conspiracy by one group of physicians to exclude others from competition.[24]

It should be noted that the Federal Trade Commission in the past has shown interest in exclusive dealing arrangements, just as it is doing in the health care industry in general. When the FTC chooses to challenge an exclusive dealing arrangement as an unfair method of competition in violation of Section 5 of the Federal Trade Commission Act, it is not necessarily constrained by all of the standards applicable to the Sherman Act or analogous state laws. Consequently, although the general type of analysis justifying exclusive departmental and closed staff arrangements should be considered as a defense if the arrangement is challenged by the FTC, the result may be somewhat less clear.[25]

Finally, further analytical considerations may arise because emerging policy developments may give a basis for the injection of new arguments on either side of the closure issue. In particular, health care providers may take advantage of the tension between the policies of the antitrust laws tending to promote competitive opportunities, and of the health planning laws toward restricting the duplication of services and avoiding excess capacity. The exclusive departmental arrangement creates a barrier to entry and forecloses otherwise available opportunities. The foreclosure may become much more significant and require more stringent analysis, as the effects of health planning reduce the availability of competitive specialized departments in a locality, and thus effectively grant some monopoly powers to physicians enjoying exclusive departmental arrangements. However, those physicians may equally well demonstrate that the arrangement tends to lower costs and therefore is favored by health planning policies as well as being prudent to fulfill the quality and coverage requirements of state law.

The prudent course in deciding to go exclusive or otherwise close a staff still appears to be to follow an extensive internal administrative procedure, evaluating all of the alternatives and the factors in favor of, as well as opposed to, a staff closure, and keeping a proper administrative record of the proceedings. However, where the objectives of the facility can be fulfilled without closing the staff entirely, serious consideration should be given to all less restrictive alternatives.

THE DENIAL OF PRIVILEGES IN AN OPEN MEDICAL STAFF

When a physician is denied privileges to join a hospital staff, either in whole or in part, the immediate impact on the individual's ability to pursue his or her profession is similar to staff privilege denials emanating from exclusive arrangements, as discussed above. The subsequent impact on the physician's reputation and practice may be even greater, however, as the individual, at least in theory, has been singled out from fellow colleagues for particularly disadvantageous treatment. If the individual denied the privileges is made unable, or substantially less able, to pursue the profession, the incentive to litigate probably is no less than that in closed staff arrangements. The potential bases for such litigation, however, are more expanded, as are the precautions and guidelines to be observed by health care facilities desiring to avoid unnecessary liability.

The most significant potential for exposure in the individual denial of privileges in an open hospital staff results from the typical method by which the decisions are made and the persons to whom the task of making the decisions (or at least highly persuasive recommendations) are delegated. In this respect, the Medicare rules of participation require that recommendations on medical staff applications be made to the governing body of the hospital by the active medical staff. The extent to which the governing body then is capable of, or inclined toward, independently analyzing and perhaps reversing recommendations of the active staff is necessarily a function of the governing body in question. Consequently, it is entirely possible that the active staff, itself composed of the potential competitors of the new applicant, actually will be capable of agreeing jointly to eliminate competition by recommending privileges be denied to the candidate. When the hospital governing body actively participates with the medical staff in a decision to deny the proposed new staff member the right to compete with the existing staff, or merely acquiesces in the staff's conduct (perhaps to avoid creating personnel controversy and dissatisfaction), the hospital itself becomes exposed to potential antitrust liability, along with the staff members.[26]

The decision to refuse staff privileges to a physician, reached in a process involving significant input by members of the medical staff and the hospital governing body, is characterized for purposes of antitrust analysis as a refusal by the institution to deal with the physician in question. Where the decision is made by a number of persons acting on behalf of multiple legal entities, it is the result of concerted action or, in antitrust parlance, a concerted refusal to deal. Although concerted refusals to deal frequently are referred to as boycotts, the term boycott may be as much a conclusion of illegality as a description of conduct and, consequently, that term is used only sparingly here.

The finding of a concert of action (requiring the participation of multiple legal entities) is the first critical point in determining the legality of a refusal to deal. Consequently, situations depending upon the participation of persons as representatives of different entities should be observed closely. Moreover, the simple decision to deny staff privileges to an individual applicant—whether by the hospital governing body individually or by a concert of action together with medical staff members—need not violate any law whatsoever. Various legal standards appear to recognize the prudence of eliminating incompetent or otherwise unqualified physicians from the marketplace. The fact that the elimination of unqualified practitioners incidentally reduces the number of physicians from whom consumers may choose to purchase services is a necessary adjunct of the process of quality control. Hospitals are required in turn to participate in this quality control process, both by direct governmental standards such as the rules on participation in the Medicare program[27] and the Joint Commission on Accreditation of Hospitals, and by the judicial expansion of the concept of negligence, which now requires that the hospital and its medical staff follow procedures to ensure that demonstrably unqualified practitioners do not injure hospital patients under the color of medical staff privileges.[28]

The important questions then become: (1) when might this quality control process result in antitrust liability for the perpetration of an illegal boycott, and (2) how can such exposure be reduced or eliminated? For the answers to these questions, consideration of the judicially developed rules on concerted refusals to deal, and the context in which the rules have been applied to health care providers, must precede the statement of conclusions that may be distilled from the cases.

Concerted Refusal To Deal Through Denial of Staff Privileges

For analytical purposes, the staff of a hospital is much like a trade association—in some instances, a peculiarly powerful trade association. The staff is composed of generally independent competitors who must perform certain joint functions in order to improve and assure the quality and reliability of the services. This joint conduct, generally quality control, concurrently should benefit the consuming public and practitioners who pass the scrutiny of their peers. The question of legal versus illegal refusal to deal in the context of formal trade associations was treated in Chapter 5. However, the question of when the denial of medical staff privileges becomes an illegal boycott involving all or part of a medical staff as well as the hospital itself is sufficiently distinct, and is treated so by the courts, to warrant independent evaluation in this chapter. This evaluation, however, first requires a brief repetition of the principles of concerted refusals to deal.

When pursued in industries other than the learned professions, concerted refusals to deal have enjoyed little, if any, tolerance from the courts. In the *Klor's* landmark 1959 case (see Chapter 1) involving a combination of manufacturers, distributors, and retailers who conspired to boycott an individual retailer, the Supreme Court held that certain restraints of trade were considered unduly restrictive in and of themselves and thus *per se* offensive against the antitrust laws. The court added succinctly that concerted refusals to deal were within this category.[29]

Over the years, as might be anticipated, courts handling cases involving concerted refusals to deal occasionally have found methods of avoiding the harsh *per se* offense treatment, as established by the Supreme Court, where the situation indicated that the consideration of justifications might be appropriate. Thus, definitions of illegal group boycotts sometimes have been narrowed in apparent efforts to allow flexibility within the law. For example, in a 1978 case a professional football player challenged the National Football League player draft as a group boycott and therefore a *per se* antitrust offense (see Chapter 1). The court ruled that although the player draft in a certain manner did constitute a concerted refusal to deal with certain players by teams not able to draft all players with whom they might otherwise desire to deal, it was not a horizontal boycott of one potential competitor by a group of other competitors. The court set guidelines that by analogy could be useful to health care providers, explaining:

> The "group boycott" designation, we believe, is properly restricted to concerted attempts by competitors to exclude horizontal competitors; it should not be applied, and has never been applied by the Supreme Court, to concerted refusals that are not designed to drive out competitors but to achieve some other goal.[30]

Medical Staff Applications of Concerted Refusals To Deal

Although numerous cases explain rules of law under which the validity of a hospital's decision to deny or revoke individual staff privileges may be analyzed, relatively few do so under antitrust principles. Changing judicial attitudes on the applicability of antitrust laws to the health care industry suggest, however, that the cases in this section should include both those determined under antitrust principles, as well as others that could have been decided on antitrust bases but were not.

If the allegations of the plaintiff in *Robinson v. Magovern*[31] are taken as true, this 1978 case presents an unusually good example of a number of the types of abuses that may occur when one group of competitors has the ability to exclude potential rivals from the marketplace. The plaintiff in this case was a thoracic surgeon who had been denied staff privileges at a hospital in Pennsylvania. He charged that the hospital, its trustees, and another thoracic surgeon had agreed to deny staff privileges in thoracic surgery to new applicants for the sole purpose of perpetuating a medical group's control of this field at the hospital. In effect, the plaintiff contended that only members of this one medical group received thoracic surgery privileges. The situation involved no formal exclusive dealing arrangement between the medical group and the hospital, and apparently there had been no hospital determination that a closed staff would improve the quality of thoracic surgery care, improve the administration of the hospital, or be preferable to the open staff that, at least in form, the facility offered to the medical community.

The differences between the two sides in *Robinson* help illustrate the difficulties that may be encountered in fixing the labels of "exclusive dealing arrangement" as opposed to "group boycott" to this type of medical staff privilege denial. The defendants contended that the situation alleged, even if true, would be only an exclusive dealing arrangement that need not violate the antitrust laws in these circumstances. The court, however, ruled that an antitrust violation existed where it was alleged that a hospital governing body in effect had extended to a medical group a veto power over new staff privilege applications, even though the veto was followed by "some procedural window dressing, including a hearing" and was used to preserve the market situation enjoyed by the favored group to the exclusion of new competition, and where the conduct substantially impaired the flow of interstate commerce (as found from contentions that the favored group received substantial Federal payments through Medicare and Medicaid programs, as would the disfavored applicant had he been allowed to practice).

The court in *Robinson* emphasized the importance of a finding that the conduct was a result of an anticompetitive motive. This can be expected to be a critical element in any antitrust action involving a denial of medical staff privileges, for even denials based solely on the basis of incompetence of the physician applicant will have an anticompetitive effect because the individual is thwarted in efforts to practice in the local market. Consequently, where anticompetitive effects can be expected even from entirely valid conduct, only the purpose of the conduct remains to be analyzed.

In addition, the court in *Robinson* afforded significant respect to nonhealth care cases that conclude that a concerted refusal to deal in itself is an antitrust violation where there is a purpose either to exclude a person or group from the market or to accomplish some other anticompetitive objective. However, the court did not enunciate clearly any conclusion that this *per se* standard would be available to the plaintiff at trial. Rather, it appeared to leave room for an interpretation that the plaintiff might be required to demonstrate a violation of the rule of reason (*i.e.*, by demonstrating that the conduct not only occurred with the illicit motive, but also had an unreasonably anticompetitive effect in the marketplace) similar to the football case described earlier.

The court's analysis in *Robinson* is interesting also for its reliance on the geographical market determinations of the local Health Systems Agency. In any rule of reason or monopolization analysis, the impact of challenged conduct must be evaluated within a definable geographic market area. Typically, establishing such a market at trial involves complex legal and economic issues that will be the subject of expert testimony and the cause of significant expense to the parties. In *Robinson*, however, the court exhibited a willingness to adopt the geographic market determinations of the HSA in its health systems plan. While such planning determinations will not always be applicable to antitrust issues, their value should not be overlooked.

The decision of the California Supreme Court in *Willis v. Santa Ana Hospital Association*,[32] discussed earlier in this chapter, illustrates a different type of anticompetitive motive that might be expected to result occasionally in the denial of medical staff privileges. In essence, the motive in question in *Willis* was not the desire simply to preserve a unique position in a hospital, but rather to dominate the practice of a certain branch of medicine in an entire geographic area. The plaintiff, a physician whose staff privileges were terminated purportedly because of questionable competence and reputation, contended that the staff privilege closure actually was the result of a conspiracy involving the hospital, certain of its directors, its administrator, and various physicians. The plaintiff also charged that this conspiracy was intended to result in the domination of the practice of medicine by osteopathic physicians and surgeons in Orange County, California, through blocking staff memberships in that county. Unlike *Robinson*, this type of situation does not lend itself to a defense of simple exclusive dealing between a hospital and a group of physicians.

The *Willis* case was decided by the California Supreme Court in 1962 when the learned professions generally were considered entirely exempt from the antitrust laws. Consequently, the court held that the challenged conduct could not have violated California state antitrust law (which, in relevant particulars, parallels federal antitrust laws). The court did find, however, that the conduct could constitute the common law tort of unreasonable interference with the plaintiff's right to pursue his lawful profession. In fact, the court's description of the nature of such a tort became the model followed by a subsequent court in the 1965 exclusive departmental challenge tested in *Blank v. Palo Alto-Stanford Medical Center* (also described earlier). Moreover, this same common law tort was described in 1975 by an Arizona court of appeals in *Datillo* (discussed on p. 153)[33] as paralleling both the Arizona state antitrust laws and the Sherman Act. In light of these later developments, the California Supreme Court's earlier decision that this situation stated a violation of the general rules prohibiting unreasonable restraints of trade, together with the court's explicit rejection of the defense that the conduct was necessary to maintain professional standards and high quality medical care, becomes of increased importance.[34]

Although medical doctors have been accused of using their professional associations to enhance their own market positions to the detriment of osteopathic physicians, this conduct ordinarily has not related directly to hospitals. A situation in which an osteopathic physician charged that the denial of staff privileges to himself and other osteopathic physicians was the result of a conspiracy between the staff medical doctors and board of trustees of that hospital was addressed, however, in *Wolf v. Jane Phillips Episcopal-Memorial Medical Cen-*

ter.[35] Although this 1975 case was dismissed for failure to allege the prerequisite impact on the flow of interstate commerce (in order to find jurisdiction under federal antitrust laws), if the court had considered the impact on the flow of reimbursement funds under Medicare and Medicaid, the outcome could well have been quite different. (The plaintiff also might have benefited from a common law tort analysis like the example established in *Willis*.)

Another method of invalidating wholesale staff privilege denials to osteopathic physicians was explained in 1958 by a Texas state court, which held that a hospital could not summarily deny privileges to persons simply because they were not graduates of schools approved by the American Medical Association. While the court considered the rule reasonable in requiring high standards of medical training, it said it was an invalid delegation of the hospital board's duty to itself determine the qualifications of its staff members.[36] Although not addressed by the court, this type of delegation creates the further danger that medical physicians in control of AMA accrediting activity could directly inhibit competition from nonmember physicians and paraprofessionals. This, in turn, could constitute an unreasonable restraint of trade.

As with the importance of demonstrating a substantial impact on interstate commerce, the importance of demonstrating the concerted (or joint) as opposed to individual nature of the challenged conduct is illustrated in *Sokol v. University Hospital, Inc.*[37] in 1975. The plaintiff contended that the denial of staff privileges in cardiac surgery was the result of a conspiracy among the hospital and others, including a cardiac surgeon, to limit the practice of such surgery at that institution to this one physician. The court's opinion does not indicate the existence of any actual exclusive dealing arrangement. The court decided that the limitation on staff privileges was a simple refusal to deal and, in the absence of a monopoly, did not violate the Sherman Act. It found that there was no agreement, combination, or conspiracy, as the action complained of was simply that of a corporation (the hospital), and the fact that the concurrence of a number of persons at the corporation caused the decision to be made would not satisfy the Sherman Act's requirement of an agreement, combination, or conspiracy.

Although this decision conforms to the rule that agents and employees of a corporation do not combine or conspire when they simply act in that capacity to reach a corporate decision, the court's analysis did not consider explicitly whether any of these persons might have been acting on their own individual behalf or in some other capacity and thereby could have fulfilled the requirement of a multiplicity of legal entities in order to find an agreement, combination, or conspiracy. By way of counter example, in *Cowan v. Gibson*,[38] a court in 1965 found that a conspiracy could have been reached between the hospital governing board and members of its medical staff to deny staff privileges to a physician. The court noted the importance of allegations that this was not simply the hospital denying staff privileges, but was a conspiracy with other physicians acting in their individual capacities. The conspiracy therefore was not simply the unilateral conduct of the hospital as a legal entity.

A variation on the theme of concerted refusal to deal with individual physicians through denial of staff privileges, and a detailed analysis of the types of rules applicable to concerted refusals to deal in the medical profession, is found in *The Feminist Women's Health Center, Inc. v. Mohammad.*[39] In this case, the plaintiff (an abortion clinic) claimed that local physicians had combined and conspired to boycott the facility, in part through the efforts of the medical staff of a nearby hospital. The court concluded that the application of standard antitrust doctrines must be harmonized with the peculiarities of the medical profession. Consequently, although the court explained that the traditional *per se* doctrine did have a certain application to medical boycotts, it allowed the defendant physicians to assert a defense based upon their bona fide concern for the public welfare.

However, where the motivation for the refusal to deal is shown to be anticompetitive in nature, and the defendants do not demonstrate their good faith efforts to preserve the quality of medical care, the plaintiff will not be required to prove that the defendants have a specific intent to restrain trade. Moreover, the court said the plaintiff might be required to demonstrate only that certain defendants acquiesced in a course of conduct, the consequences of which would be to restrain trade, and that anticompetitive intent might be inferred from that acquiescence.[40]

Considerations for Prospective Conduct

A majority of challenges to staff privilege denials historically have been pursued under constitutional or statutory principles requiring fair hearings and decisions pursuant to certain reasonably objective standards. The tensions and difficulties created for the conduct of health care providers in reaching staff privilege recommendations and decisions with the concurrent requirements of making qualitative evaluations to meet the standard of care required to avoid malpractice liability, while holding hearings and reaching decisions under written objective standards in order to meet due process and Medicare (as well as probable state law) requirements, suggest a significant part of the answer to the potential antitrust problems present in the selection of medical staffs.

In other industries where self-regulation is required by statute, the otherwise clear application of antitrust principles may give way to allow the proper fulfillment of the self-regulation mandate. The statutory requirement that stock exchanges, for example, establish rules that are just and adequate to ensure fair dealing and to protect investors requires that the exchanges engage in self-regulation, involving in part the disciplining of members who violate the rules. Where such self-regulation is required by federal law, there is an implied repeal of the antitrust laws to the extent necessary to allow the proper conduct of this process. Similarly, where self-regulation is required by state law, a state action defense may be raised.

The self-regulation process can transform an otherwise clearly violative group boycott into an issue of whether the particular act of self-regulation was justified in the circumstances. Where it was justified, the antitrust laws could hardly apply. Where it was not, the specter of antitrust enforcement is raised again.[41] The hospital and its medical staff thus face the continuing dilemma of fulfilling their self-regulation duties in a justifiable manner that will not exceed the scope of their proper powers or constitute the pursuit of anticompetitive motives. However, where medical staff decisions are made under all of the rules in the Code of Federal Regulations or by the Joint Commission on Accreditation of Hospitals, where due process rights are observed, and where staff privilege denials are made to improve or assure the quality of care and not to exclude competitors from the market, then the self-regulation process would appear to be working, and antitrust principles, to that extent, would be inapplicable.

NOTES

1. 234 Cal.App.2d 377, 44 Cal.Rptr. 572.

2. 58 Cal.2d 806 (1962).

3. Because of *Goldfarb* (note 47, Chapter 1), the applicability of this part of the holding in *Willis* is doubtful today.

4. 246 Cal.App.2d 673, 55 Cal.Rptr. 118 (1966).

5. 82 Cal.App.3d 368 (1978).

6. 82 Cal.App.3d at 385.

7. 82 Cal.App.3d at 388.

8. The court did note that a balancing test is appropriate in determining whether the interference with the pursuit of a trade or calling is unreasonable. This court weighs the respective importance to society and the parties, on the one hand, of protecting the activities interfered with and, on the other hand, permitting the interference. The court said the factors to be considered include the nature of the acts or conduct, the objects thought to be accomplished and the interest thought to be advanced by the acts or conduct, and the extent of tł hardship caused to the person against whom the acts or conduct is directed. Rather than actually perform the balancing, however, the court held that the executive committee of the medical staff of the hospital had performed this balancing act and had determined that a closed staff operation was preferable. The court did not purport to balance all the factors itself, but decided only that the balancing performed by the executive committee was not arbitrary or capricious. *See,* 82 Cal.App.3d at 394.

9. 23 Ariz.App. 392, 533 P.2d 700, 74 ALR 3d 1259 (1975).

10. 226 S.W.2d 908 (Texas App. 1950).

11. 522 F.2d 1133 (4th Cir. 1975).

12. 104 N.W.2d 633 (S.Ct. Minn. 1960).

13. The court in *Benell* further warns, quite validly, that individual state statutes must be checked in determining whether the conduct of a public hospital violates such statutes. *See*, 104 N.W.2d at 637.

14. Florida App., 205 So.2d 11 (1967).

15. 453 Pennsylvania 60, 311 A.2d 634 (1973).

16. 368 A.2d 334 (N.J. 1976).

17. *Davis v. Morristown Memorial Hosp.*, 254 A.2d (N.J. Super.Ct. 1969).

18. *Walsky v. Pascack Valley Hosp.*, 367 A.2d 1204 (N.J. Super.Ct. 1976).

19. *See* description of the *Goldfarb* case in Chapter 1.

20. *See e.g., Zamiri v. William Beaumont Hosp.* 430 F.Supp. 875 (E.D. Mich. 1977), where the court held that if a single physician could demonstrate that a significant portion of his income would have been gained from federal programs such as Medicare, then the restriction upon his ability to practice could be demonstrated to have the requisite impact on interstate commerce.

21. 521 F.2d 1230 (3rd Cir. 1975).

22. The enforceability of a covenant not to compete is often affected by state statutes. A Florida state court has held a two-year postterm covenant not to compete to be enforceable in the contract of a physicians' partnership. In essence, where any physician withdrew from the partnership, that individual was prohibited from practicing in that county for two years. *Chessick Clinic, P.A. v. Jones*, Trade Cases (CCH) ¶ 62,435 (Fla.App. 1979).

23. 246 U.S. 231, 238, 38 S.Ct. 242, 244 (1918). *See* description of guidelines established by this case in Chapter 1.

24. *See, e.g., United States v. Topco Associates, Inc.*, 405 U.S. 596, 92 S.Ct.Rptr. 1126 (1972), where the court found that a group purchasing association, owned and controlled by a group of members who otherwise were competitors in a grocery store market, had been used by its owners as a vehicle for the division of markets, thus constituting a horizontal conspiracy in restraint of trade. *See* also, the discussion in *American Motor Inns, Inc. v. Holiday Inns*, 521 F.2d at 1242 (*supra*, note 21), explaining that where the parent franchisor of the various Holiday Inn motels that was used as a vehicle through which the horizontally competitive franchisee motels could veto the development of those that would be competitively situated with existing ones, it similarly would constitute a horizontal market allocation and a violation of the Sherman Act.

25. *See, e.g., Fashion Originators' Guild of Am., Inc. v. Federal Trade Commission*, 312 U.S. 457 (1941), explaining that the Federal Trade Commission Act reaches incipient combinations, such as the scheme there challenged where the sale of textiles was made only on the condition that the buyers not deal in textiles copied from other sellers' designs. *Federal Trade Commission v. Motion Picture Advertising Serv. Co.*, 344 U.S. 392, 73 S.Ct. 361 (1953), where the court explained that the Federal Trade Commission Act reaches unfair methods of competition, even beyond those illegal under other antitrust statutes or common law. Notably, the result in the *Motion Picture Advertising* case was not to invalidate entirely the exclusive contracts there challenged but to limit the length of the term of those contracts to one year.

26. *See, Interstate Circuit, Inc. v. United States*, 306 U.S. 208, 59 S.Ct. 467 (1939) demonstrating that acquiescence in a course of conduct, the necessary consequence of which would be to restrain trade, is sufficient to imply intent and to establish a conspiracy.

27. 20 CFR 405.1023.

28. *See, e.g., Joiner v. Mitchell County Hosp. Auth. et al.*, 125 Ga.App.1, 186 SE 2d 307, 51 ALR. 3d 976, recognizing a duty of due care on the part of the hospital in selecting staff physicians; *Corleto v. Shore Memorial Hosp.*, 138 N.J. Super.Ct. 302, 358. A.2d 534 (1976), permitting a malpractice suit against an entire hospital medical staff on the theory that the staff shared some responsibility for the quality of those practitioners with privileges.

29. *Klor's, Inc. v. Broadway-Hale Stores, Inc.*, 359 U.S. 207, 212, 79 S.Ct. 705, 709 (1959).

30. *Smith v. Pro Football, Inc.*, 1978—2 Trade Cases (CCH) ¶ 62,338, 76,031–76,034.

31. 456 F.Supp. 1000 (W.D. Pa. 1978).

32. 58 Cal.2d 806, 26 Cal.Rptr. 640, 376 P.2d 578 (1962).

33. *Datillo v. Tucson Gen. Hosp.*, *supra*, note 9.

34. The court in *Willis* explained: "We reject the suggestion that, in order to maintain professional standards and medical care of high quality, private hospitals and their staffs must have absolute discretion to exclude doctors from membership, without the possibility of a suit for damages resulting from the exclusion. The burden of defending suits cannot warrant denial of relief to one injured by wholly unjustifiable conduct such as is alleged in the present case." 58 Cal.2d at 810–11.

35. 513 F.2d 684 (10 Cir. 1975).

36. *Duson v. Poage*, 318 S.W.2d 89 (1958); a similar result was reached in *Greisman v. Newcomb Hosp.*, 192 A.2d 817 (N.J. Super.Ct. 1963).

37. 402 F.Supp. 1029 (D. Mass. 1975).

38. 392 S.W.2d 307 (Mo. 1965).

39. 415 F.Supp. 1258 (N.D. Fla. 1976), *rev'd on other grounds*, 586 F.2d 530 (5th Cir. 1978).

40. 415 F.Supp. at 1267.

41. *See, Silver v. NYSE*, 373 U.S. 341, 83 S.Ct. 1246 (1963).

Chapter 7

Relations With Health Insurers

While health care providers have become ever more dependent upon payments from insurers for services to patients, insurers have become correspondingly more involved in the daily economic affairs of providers. In fact, with the development of Blue Cross and Blue Shield programs, and more recently of Health Maintenance Organizations and other prepaid health plans, the distinction between the business of a provider and the business of an insurer has become increasingly vague. As insurers have become involved in the establishment of provider charges and even in decisions of quantity and type of care to be supplied, providers concurrently have become involved in self-insurance, prepaid health plans, and other risk-spreading programs.

ANTITRUST EXEMPTION FOR THE BUSINESS OF INSURANCE

These trends notwithstanding, nominal distinctions between providers and insurers generally have been maintained, and the working relationships continue to be important to all parties. Of increasing importance, however, is the concern over the extent to which insurers' efforts to improve their own industry performance or market positions can be allowed to impact adversely upon individual providers or related entities. Insurers have proved capable, for example, of arranging payment programs that discriminate against nonphysician practitioners or against physicians who are not members of preferred groups. Similarly, insurance arrangements may work to the disadvantage of individual institutional providers that fail to qualify for, or could not economically survive with, certain contracts. Agreements between certain providers and insurers also may directly disadvantage other providers or even other insurers.

The potential for restraints of trade emanating from the conduct of insurers or the joint conduct of insurers and providers, then, is apparent. Influence over the pricing mechanism (price fixing), concerted refusals to deal, and attempted or actual monopolization of markets all are possible outcomes of relationships with insurers. The application of the antitrust laws to insurers, however, is complicated by a statutory exemption, the McCarran-Ferguson Act (hereinafter the McCarran Act),[1] which specifically exempts from antitrust scrutiny the "business of insurance" to the extent it is regulated by state law. The McCarran Act exemption does not, however, immunize conduct in the business of insurance that amounts to a boycott, coercion, or intimidation.

Because of the McCarran Act exemption, it is particularly important to analyze restraints of trade that result from relationships with insurers, to attempt to understand when the conduct of an insurer is not necessarily the business of insurance (a phrase of ever-narrowing scope), when the business of insurance is not regulated adequately by state law for the exemption to operate, when the business of insurance results in a boycott, coercion, or intimidation that causes the loss of the exemption, and when the conduct of a provider in conjunction with an insurer may result in liability for one or both of the parties.

BACKGROUND OF THE INSURANCE EXEMPTION

From the adoption of the Sherman Act in 1890, and continuing until 1944, there existed a universal understanding that the sale of an insurance policy did not constitute interstate commerce and, therefore, that insurance was beyond the scope of federal antitrust laws. However, the Supreme Court in 1944 departed from this 54-year precedent in the landmark case of *United States v. South-Eastern Underwriters Association*, in which it ruled that the business of insurance was interstate commerce and that the Congress that had enacted the Sherman Act had not intended to exempt the insurance industry from the antitrust laws.[2]

Within a year after that decision, Congress enacted the McCarran-Ferguson Act, essentially reestablishing a portion of the previously total exemption enjoyed by insurance companies. As the intended scope and legislative history of the McCarran Act has become a matter of significant concern in recent Supreme Court decisions interpreting and applying the act, legislative events relating to its adoption deserve special consideration. In general, the Supreme Court has inferred subsequently from the legislative history of the McCarran Act that the primary concern of Congress in adopting this measure was to insure the states' continued ability to tax and regulate the business of insurance.[3] The antitrust exemption was of only secondary concern.

The legislative history of the act demonstrates a Congressional recognition that it is difficult to provide insurance, in the sense of underwriting risks, without cooperation among various insurance companies. Thus, the primary concern of those who adopted the act, with respect to antitrust applications in the insurance industry, was that cooperative rate-making mechanisms should enjoy an antitrust exemption. The Supreme Court itself recognized the importance of the congressional concern for allowing cooperative rate-making efforts, in part because of a study prepared by the National Association of Insurance Commissioners and submitted to Congress before the adoption of the McCarran Act. Based upon this study, a Senate committee concluded:

> For these and other reasons the subcommittee believes it would be a mistake to permit or require the unrestricted competition contemplated by the antitrust laws to apply to the insurance business. To prohibit combined efforts for statistical and rate-making purposes would be a backwards step in the development of a progressive business.[4]

The anticipated nature of the exempted rate-making effort was further explained by Senator Homer Ferguson, a coauthor of the bill, who explained the purpose as follows:

> This bill would permit—and I think it is fair to say that it is intended to permit—rating bureaus, because in the last session we passed a bill for the District of Columbia allowing rating. What we saw as wrong was the fixing of rates without statutory authority in the states; but we believe that State rights should permit a State to say that it believes in a rating bureau. I think the insurance companies have convinced many members of the legislature that we cannot have open competition in fixing rates on insurance. If we do, we shall have chaos. There will be failures, and failures always follow losses.[5]

Congressional discussion of the McCarran Act thus assumed a protective quality, visualizing state-regulated rate-setting bureaus to avoid failures among insurance companies that otherwise might be driven to set rates at levels inadequate to protect and assure the viability of the insurer. In addition, data dissemination in a manner adequate to allow the formulation of rates in full light of the experiences of all members of the industry was to be protected, even though the data dissemination necessarily would influence the pricing mechanism. The legislative discussions of the proposed exemption did not, however, indicate an intention to protect overtly predatory conduct by insurers who might seek to eliminate rivals, nor to offer some unique protection to insurance companies that choose to diversify into, or otherwise profit from, other industries.

The statute that emerged from these Congressional considerations, however, was somewhat less detailed than some had suggested,[6] and offered language that could be, and has been, interpreted in various ways. The relevant operative antitrust exemption reads as follows:

. . . after June 30, 1948, the Act of July 2, 1890, as amended, known as the Sherman Act, and the Act of October 15, 1914, as amended, known as the Clayton Act, and the Act of September 26, 1914, known as the Federal Trade Commission Act, as amended, shall be applicable to the business of insurance to the extent that such business is not regulated by State law.[7]

The following specific exception from the antitrust exemption also was provided:

Nothing contained in this chapter shall render the said Sherman Act inapplicable to any agreement to boycott, coerce, or intimidate, or act of boycott, coercion, or intimidation.[8]

To reach the conclusion that the McCarran Act exemption protects any particular conduct from antitrust scrutiny thus requires finding first that the conduct: (1) constitutes the business of insurance; (2) is regulated by state law; and (3) does not constitute a boycott, coercion, or intimidation. The courts applying this exemption, particularly to conduct in or affecting the health care industry, have used vastly different tests and definitions and consequently have reached quite different results on various occasions. Not until early 1979 did the Supreme Court offer detailed guidance on the scope of the McCarran Act exemption. The ensuing consideration of the scope of this exemption, therefore, focuses primarily on the Supreme Court's guidance, with references to assistance and analogies in lower court decisions.

THE MEANING OF 'THE BUSINESS OF INSURANCE'

The Supreme Court early in 1979 explained in detail the scope of the exemption for the "business of insurance" in its long-awaited decision in *Group Life and Health Insurance Company v. Royal Drug Company*.[9] The plaintiffs in the *Royal Drug* case were 18 owners of independent pharmacies in the San Antonio, Texas, area. The pharmacy owners sued the Group Life and Health Insurance Company, also known as Blue Shield of Texas, and three other local pharmacies. The plaintiffs contended that Blue Shield had entered into agreements with other pharmacies (including the three defendant entities) that served to fix the retail price of drugs and caused Blue Shield policyholders not to purchase drugs from the plaintiffs. The federal trial court had dismissed the action, concluding that the challenged agreements constituted the "business of insurance," were regulated by the state of Texas, and were not boycotts and therefore were exempted from antitrust scrutiny under the McCarran Act. The Supreme Court, however, concluded that the challenged arrangements were not a part of the "business of insurance," and therefore were not entitled to McCarran Act protection.

The Supreme Court said the challenged arrangements worked essentially as follows: Blue Shield offers insurance policies to consumers. One of the benefits is that policyholders are entitled to obtain prescription drugs, subject only to a certain deductible amount for each purchase. To provide these drugs to its policyholders, Blue Shield offers to enter into "pharmacy agreements" with any and all pharmacies that choose to participate. At pharmacies that do participate, Blue Shield policyholders may purchase drugs simply by paying $2 per purchase to the pharmacy, and no further amounts. The pharmacy is reimbursed by Blue Shield for its actual cost of drugs sold, and keeps the $2 cash payment from the policyholder as its profit on the transaction. The policyholder is presented with a very different transaction, however, in dealing with pharmacies that are not participants in the Blue Shield agreements. At these latter pharmacies, the policyholder must pay the pharmacy the full price of the drug, then submit the bill to Blue Shield for reimbursement. The policyholder is reimbursed by Blue Shield for only 75 percent of the difference between $2 and the price of the drug.

The plaintiffs contended that smaller independent pharmacies, themselves included, could not afford to distribute prescription drugs for the $2 gross "profit" offered by Blue Shield, and therefore were economically prohibited from participating in the program. They concluded from these facts that the Blue Shield program constituted a form of price fixing in the providing of prescription drugs to consumers and that it caused most policyholders to deal only with pharmacies that did participate in the agreements. They charged that only by dealing with such pharmacies were the policyholders spared the nuisance of applying for reimbursement from Blue Shield, while policyholders who dealt with the plaintiffs were at an economic disadvantage because they were reimbursed for only 75 percent of their expenditures in excess of $2. The plaintiffs contended that this arrangement constituted an unreasonable restraint of trade in violation of the Sherman Act. Blue Shield replied that, aside from not violating the Sherman Act, the conduct was part of the business of insurance and was exempted from Sherman Act consideration pursuant to the McCarran Act. While the Supreme Court did not reach the question of whether the conduct would violate the Sherman Act (this question being saved for a federal trial court to consider later), it analyzed the meaning of "business of insurance" extensively and, for the first time, offered a definition to help remedy the previous conflict between different definitions then being applied by courts in various parts of the country.

The court said the statute exempted from antitrust scrutiny only the "business of insurance," not the business of insurance companies in general. Consequently, the mere fact that the conduct in question was perpetrated by an insurance company was not sufficient to invoke the protection of the McCarran Act. Second, the court determined that certain types of arrangements could be regulated by state insurance commissioners under state law, and did not constitute the "business of insurance" for purposes of the McCarran Act. A leading example of this situation is the variable annuity life insurance policy, whereby subscribers pay fixed amounts to the insurance company and in return receive a lifetime annuity whose value rises and falls with the quality of the investment decisions made by the insurance company. Although these policies may be offered by insurance companies and may be regulated by insurance commissioners, the court held, an annuity of this type was not the "business of insurance."

The court ruled that the critical element in the "business of insurance" was the underwriting or spreading of risk. It adopted the following language from an insurance commentator:

> It is the characteristic of insurance that a number of risks are accepted, some of which involve losses, and that such losses are spread over all the risks so as to enable the insurer to accept each risk at a slight fraction of the possible liability upon it.[10]

The court held that the Blue Shield arrangements did not constitute the "business of insurance" because they did not involve any underwriting or spreading of risk. Rather, it said, the arrangements merely were agreements for the purchases of goods and services by Blue Shield from the participating pharmacies. Although the agreements allowed Blue Shield to reduce the cost of its goods purchased, and thereby to reduce the price of policies to policyholders, this did not constitute the "business of insurance." In essence, the court found these arrangements were similar to any other type of arrangements by insurance companies in their efforts to keep down costs, which necessarily would impact upon insurance rates. A most extreme example offered by the court was a hypothetical situation in which an insurance company might determine that the best way to keep down the cost of drugs to policyholders would be simply to acquire a chain of drugstores. The court said such an acquisition, although helping to hold down the price of policies, would not constitute the "business of insurance."

The court did agree that the "business of insurance" included, beyond the function of spreading risk, the relationship between the insurer and the insured in the form of the insurance contract. This relationship included the type of policy that could be issued, its reliability, and its interpretation and enforcement—all those being elements of the "business of insurance." In the Blue Shield situation, however, the court said the links between the plan and the pharmacies were not agreements or relationships between the insurer and the insured; the merely incidental fact that the agreements helped to hold down prices of insurance policies did not make them part of the relationship between the insurer and the insured.

Of particular importance to health maintenance organizations and other prepaid health plans was the court's long description of the background and reasons for its conclusion that health care plans, even though they might achieve a certain risk spreading by providing variable amounts of service at a fixed cost, did not constitute the "business of insurance" for purposes of McCarran Act protection, notwithstanding potential state regulation by insurance commissioners. The court analogized prepaid health care plans to the Blue Shield pharmacy agreements, and adopted the following language, essentially describing all such arrangements as bulk purchases of health care services rather than as contracts to accept and spread risk:

> Whether the contract is insurance or indemnity there must be a risk of loss to which one party may be subjected by contingent or future events and an assumption of it by legally binding arrangement with another. Even the most loosely stated conceptions of insurance require these elements. Hazard is essential and so is a shifting of its incidence. . . .
>
> Although Group Health's activities may be considered in one aspect as creating security against loss from illness or accident, more truly they constitute the quantity purchase of well-rounded, continuous medical service by its members. Group Health is in fact and in function a consumer cooperative. The functions of such an organization are not identical with those of insurance or indemnity companies. The latter are concerned primarily, if not exclusively with risk. . . . On the other hand, the cooperative is concerned principally with *getting services to its members* and doing so at lower prices made possible by quantity purchasing and economics in operation.[11]

In the *Royal Drug* case, the Supreme Court thus adopted a very narrow interpretation of the meaning of "business of insurance," excluding many of the activities of Blue Cross and Blue Shield organizations as well as the primary functions of prepaid health care plans. The *Royal Drug* opinion invalidated numerous lower court decisions that had adopted a broad interpretation of "business of insurance"[12] as recently as 1977.

Although it may be understood now that the conduct of insurance companies that relates directly to providing supplies or services to policyholders is not a part of the "business of insurance" for purposes of the McCarran Act antitrust exemption, a still valid example of conduct that is a part of the "business of insurance" was analyzed by the Supreme Court only a few months before the *Royal Drug* decision. In 1978, in *St. Paul Fire and Marine Insurance Company v. Barry*,[13] (which is discussed in detail in the section on boycotts later in this chapter) the court thus appeared to assume that an agreement among four local insurance companies, in which three of the four agreed to refuse to deal with policyholders of the fourth, fell within the meaning of the McCarran Act term "business of insurance." Presumably, such an agreement involves the relationship between insurer and insured, meaning in essence simply a joint agreement not to issue certain insurance policies.

Examples of insurance-related conduct previously thought exempt under the McCarran Act, but now clearly beyond the scope of the exemption, include certain California prepaid dental care plans as analyzed by a federal trial court in a 1976 case titled *Manasen v. California Dental Services.*[14]

In this instance, 11 dentists sued a corporation engaged in the administration and operation of prepaid dental care plans, contending that the defendants had conspired to fix fees and had monopolized the California prepaid dental care market. The trial court granted a judgment for the defendants, explaining that the company was engaged in the business of insurance and therefore was exempted from antitrust scrutiny under the McCarran Act. The defendant was not even licensed by the State Department of Insurance and was not regulated under the State Insurance Code. The court concluded, nevertheless, that the "business of insurance" could embrace arrangements that did not involve actual insurance companies, and that activities that had a substantial effect on rate making, including settlement of claims, limitation of costs, and payments to service providers, were part of the "business of insurance."

Similarly, many prepaid health care plans had been determined previously to fall within the meaning of the McCarran Act "business of insurance" exemption.[15] The antitrust exemption previously enjoyed by many Blue Shield, Blue Cross, and prepaid health care plans no longer can be anticipated, however, and even traditional insurance companies must expect to receive ordinary antitrust scrutiny when they engage in conduct beyond that now narrowly defined as the "business of insurance."

STATE REGULATION

A finding that challenged conduct is a part of the "business of insurance" is not in itself sufficient to invoke the antitrust exemption of the McCarran Act. The act explicitly provides that the antitrust laws are not applicable to the business of insurance only ". . . to the extent that such business is not regulated by State law." Consequently, to invoke the McCarran Act's protection it is necessary to find that the challenged conduct was regulated by state law.

The Supreme Court has not yet explicitly addressed the question of the scope of the McCarran Act phrase "regulated by State law." Lower courts, however, generally have applied relatively relaxed standards, and this particular requisite of McCarran Act immunity has not presented difficulties for most defendants.

In the *Manasen* case described on p. 180, for example, the same federal trial court that defined the "business of insurance" so broadly adopted a very lenient approach in determining the existence and adequacy of state regulation. Although it was undisputed in that case that the State Insurance Commissioner took no part in regulating the actual conduct in issue, the court applied a rule of such breadth that virtually any state regulation of the business of insurance was adequate to invoke the McCarran Act protection for any conduct in that business. The court specifically explained that the McCarran Act exemption did not require a finding of conflict between the federal antitrust laws and state regulation or that the state scheme of regulation actually was being enforced. The mere existence of regulatory statutes capable of being enforced, it said, was sufficient to invoke the McCarran Act protection. The court commented that even state antitrust laws applicable to insurance could be considered adequate to invoke that protection.

The court in *Manasen* looked to language of the Fifth Circuit Court of Appeals, although the 1975 case upon which it relied applied a somewhat less broad or middle ground, standard. This latter case, *Crawford v. American Title Insurance Company*,[16] involved charges of a combination and conspiracy to fix and maintain premiums charged for the issuance of title insurance in a certain area as well as alleged monopolization of this part of commerce. The defendants contended that the McCarran Act exempted their conduct from antitrust scrutiny. The plaintiffs argued, however, that although the activity was in fact the business of insurance, the specific conduct alleged had not been regulated by the state. The court ruled that the very conduct in issue was subject to regulation by the State Insurance Commissioner. The court did not attempt specifically to determine whether application of the antitrust laws to this conduct was somehow inconsistent with or repugnant to the state insurance regulation, nor did it decide whether the State Insurance Commissioner actually had passed upon the conduct as opposed to merely having the power to do so had he so chosen. Nevertheless, the court held that the McCarran Act exempted the alleged price fixing and monopolization from antitrust scrutiny.

The relatively relaxed standard for determining whether state regulation is adequate to fulfill the requirements for McCarran Act protection, as exemplified by the cases described above, appears to be a valid rule so far. In fact, when the Fifth Circuit Court of Appeals issued its decision in the *Royal Drug* case (later affirmed by the Supreme Court), it discussed the *Crawford* ruling and did not question the reasoning of the court in that earlier case.[17] When the Supreme Court later affirmed the *Royal Drug* case, it did not discuss the Fifth Circuit's apparent acceptance of the *Crawford* standard. Lest too much be made of this point, it should be noted that the Supreme Court found the conduct in question to be beyond the scope of the McCarran Act exemption without reaching the state regulation issue. Consequently, the court was by no means specifically validating the *Crawford* standard.

At least one commentator has suggested that the McCarran Act standard of exempting the business of insurance only to the extent that it is regulated by state law should be interpreted to exempt it only where the application of the antitrust laws actually conflicts with the state regulatory scheme.[18] Such an approach appears to be consistent with the general application of the state action doctrine, as limited by decisions such as the *Goldfarb* and *Cantor* cases discussed earlier, and also is consistent with the general policy of construing antitrust exemptions narrowly. It also is possible that, because of the narrow construction of the meaning of the phrase "business of insurance" by the Supreme Court in *Royal Drug,* such an approach no longer would significantly reduce the effective exemption conferred by the McCarran Act.

In addition, there is at least some indication in the legislative history of the McCarran Act to the effect that its antitrust exemption was in essence a validation of the doctrine of *Parker v. Brown* as applied to state action in the insurance industry.[19] If the McCarran exemption is taken this narrowly, however, it raises the additional question of the extent to which state action was intended to confer antitrust immunity in the absence of specific enabling legislation such as the McCarran Act or the Agricultural Marketing Act involved in the *Parker v. Brown* case (which first explained this exemption) itself.

At this point, however, there still is some variation in the approaches taken by lower courts to determine the extent of state regulation required to allow the insurer in an antitrust action to rely upon the McCarran Act defense. In most instances, the state regulation aspect of this defense has been construed liberally by the courts.[20]

BOYCOTTS, COERCION AND INTIMIDATION

Even where challenged conduct is determined to be a part of the business of insurance and is regulated adequately by state law, the McCarran Act exemption is specifically inapplicable where the conduct constitutes an agreement to boycott, coerce, or intimidate, or an act of boycott, coercion, or intimidation.[21]

As with the other portions of the McCarran Act, the meaning of this section has produced diverse opinions and various forms of speculation as to its intended breadth. In June 1978, however, the Supreme Court issued a detailed opinion on this issue, offering significant guidance for those who might become concerned with the scope of this exception from the otherwise available antitrust exemption. Thus, in *St. Paul Fire and Marine Insurance Company v. Barry,*[22] the court addressed an alleged conspiracy among the only four insurance companies selling medical malpractice insurance in Rhode Island. The plaintiffs were a group of physicians and their patients. They contended that when one of the four carriers changed its policy approach from a "claims made" type to an "occurrence" basis, it attempted to force the physicians in the state to go along with the change by obtaining the agreement of the three other carriers that they would not do business with policyholders of this fourth carrier if the policyholders attempted to switch carriers to avoid the new requirement of insuring on the "occurrence" basis. The plaintiffs charged that the insurance companies also engaged in an agreement to discriminate in rates and to fix prices, as well as a collective refusal to deal.

The trial court concluded that the challenged conduct was exempted from antitrust scrutiny pursuant to the McCarran Act, as the boycott exception was not then interpreted to refer to conduct by insurers that disadvantaged policyholders. Rather, the trial court concluded (as had numerous other courts at that time) that the boycott exception referred only to conduct among insurance companies against other insurance companies or against insurance agents. The Supreme Court, however, held that the boycott exception had a broader meaning, explaining that the generic concept of boycott referred to a method of pressuring a party with whom one had a dispute by withholding, or enlisting others to withhold, patronage or services from the target.

The court considered the cases and commentary that distinguished concerted refusals to deal that warranted *per se* invalidation from refusals to deal that were not inherently destructive of competition and therefore were analyzed under the rule of reason standards. The court held that the difference between a concerted refusal to deal that was *per se* invalid and one that could be tested under the rule of reason was not the issue with respect to the McCarran Act exception. Rather, it said, any concerted refusal to deal could be considered a boycott sufficient to remove the challenged conduct from the otherwise available McCarran Act exemption. Consequently, although the court did not expressly question the reasoning of the Sherman Act boycott cases that depended upon the conclusion that some concerted refusals to deal were not boycotts and therefore not *per se* invalid, it did suggest a new line of explanation in those boycott cases. Perhaps the term boycott in the future no longer will indicate a conclusion that certain conduct is *per se* invalid but, rather, will be only the beginning of the analysis to determine the legality of challenged refusals to deal.

As for the conduct of the four insurance companies in the *Barry* case, the Supreme Court held that the conduct might be characterized with various language but, in any event, could fairly be viewed as "an organized boycott" of one insurer's policyholders. It said the boycott was being undertaken solely to force the physician policyholders and certain hospital policyholders to agree to a significant curtailment of the coverage they had enjoyed previously. The insurer thus seeking to curtail coverage, the court added, had succeeded in enlisting the assistance of the three rival insurance competitors, thus forming a conspiracy and combination to prevent any of the competitors from dealing with certain policyholders. The court held quite simply that the term boycott as used in the McCarran Act was not limited to concerted activity against insurance companies or agents or even against competitors of members of the boycotting group.

Although the Supreme Court in *Barry* appeared at first to apply a definition of boycott that would encompass any concerted refusal to deal, it did carve out an area of potential refusals to deal that were specifically not addressed in this case. The court emphasized that the conduct occurred outside of the regulatory or cooperative arrangements established by the Rhode Island insurance laws. The state had not authorized the conduct in question, the court said, and the insurance laws did not require or otherwise authorize the concerted refusal to deal with the customers of one insurance company. Rather, it found that the boycott was entirely a private agreement in the form of an attempt at regulation by a private combination of insurance companies. The court said the situation did not involve the allocation of risks in a particular fashion pursuant to state regulatory policy, nor was there any indication that the declination to insure particular risks could have been made on the basis of state policy to avoid undermining other regulatory goals, such as the assurance of solvency of the insurance companies.

The court thus explicitly avoided a conclusion that the boycott exception from McCarran Act protection reached all concerted activity among insurance companies, and preserved the *Parker v. Brown* state action doctrine as potentially protecting the action required of insurance companies under state regulatory authority, even where that conduct otherwise would fall outside of McCarran Act protection.

The significance of the *Barry* decision is exemplified by the contrasting approaches taken by other courts, which had concluded previously that the McCarran Act boycott exception allowed antitrust actions against insurers only where the boycotts took the form of blacklists by groups of insurance companies against other insurance firms, or similar horizontal conduct. In *Doctors, Inc. v. Blue Cross of Greater Philadelphia*,[23] for example, a federal court of appeals in 1976 disallowed an action by a hospital against a hospitalization insurer and a health planning agency. The hospital had alleged that the defendants had perpetrated a concerted refusal to deal with the plaintiff hospital and had induced a group boycott against the plaintiff by certain patients. The court found that there was no boycott, coercion, or intimidation in this situation.

Although this opinion conformed to earlier analyses of limiting the McCarran Act boycott exception to action taken against insurance companies, the decision in *Barry* now indicates this type of concerted refusal to deal directed against a hospital could equally be considered a boycott under the McCarran Act exception.

The Supreme Court's decision in *Barry* further validates the approach taken by lower courts that earlier had attempted to use the boycott exception as one means of narrowing the antitrust immunity offered by the McCarran Act. A 1978 example of the application of this general approach, allowing broader use of the antitrust laws in the insurance context, is in *Carl Bartholomew v. Virginia Chiropractors Association*,[24] where the plaintiff chiropractor charged that certain insurers had conspired with state and national chiropractic associations to fix prices and boycott certain chiropractors. Although the conduct was assumed to fall within the "business of insurance," a broad reading of the boycott exception allowed the prosecution of an antitrust action.

The chiropractic portion of the health services industry also was involved in the 1976 decision in *Ballard v. Blue Shield of Southern W. Va., Inc.*,[25] where the chiropractors alleged that certain physicians, medical associations, and others, had combined and conspired to cause a refusal of health insurance for chiropractic services. The plaintiffs charged that this conduct restrained and monopolized the distribution of health services and health insurance by making chiropractic services financially unattractive to patients, while the services of medical doctors became relatively more attractive, although without the disparate insurance treatment these latter services would be more expensive. Although the plaintiffs had not used the term boycott in describing the challenged conduct, the court applied the broad interpretation of the McCarran Act and concluded that the allegations did charge a group boycott in violation of the Sherman Act and, therefore, also fell within this exception from McCarran Act protection. Consequently, this Sherman Act case against the insurance companies, medical association, and individual physicians was cognizable.

It appears unlikely now that the boycott exception from McCarran Act protection can be read so narrowly as to permit protection of private activities of insurance companies, associations, or groups of physicians or other practitioners, to exclude or disadvantage competitors, whether those competitors be other insurance companies, other physicians, hospitals, or otherwise. Moreover, activities jointly undertaken to exclude insurance policyholders from otherwise available market opportunities are unlikely to be protected by the McCarran Act.

FUTURE DEVELOPMENTS OF THE INSURANCE EXEMPTION

The National Commission for the Review of Antitrust Laws and Procedures has completed its studies and issued recommendations for modification of the antitrust laws, particularly in the area of exemptions. These suggestions are being incorporated in legislation submitted to Congress and could well influence the future of the McCarran Act exemption.

As for the insurance industry, the commission acknowledged a continuing need for insurers to receive accurate information based on credible data in order to estimate future losses and set their premium rates. The commission, however, criticized the broad grant of immunity applied by the courts under the McCarran Act, concluding that this immunity had gone beyond the original legislative purpose of permitting state regulatory mechanisms to function without federal intervention, rather than to give the industry a broad license to operate without antitrust scrutiny. In its Report to the President and the Attorney General, the commission even used this highly critical language:

> This indiscriminate immunity is granted whether or not the practice is necessary for the effective functioning of the insurance industry, the improvement of the insurance product, or the fulfillment of state regulatory goals; whether or not the practice is condoned, authorized or punished by state authorities; and whether or not it is anticompetitive or anti-consumer.[26]

The commission concluded that it could find little, if any, evidence in favor of the present breadth of the insurance immunity. To the contrary, it recommended that Congress adopt legislation specifying behavior that would be lawful for antitrust purposes in effecting a transition from its previously exempt status to that of an industry where antitrust principles were applicable, consistent with general principles of federalism.

Generally consistent with the approach taken by the President's commission, both the Department of Justice and the Federal Trade Commission began exploring issues involving the McCarran Act exemption, including relationships between hospitals and insurers. It is entirely possible that present reimbursement mechanisms, creating various exclusive relationships between insurers and health care providers, will be the subject of future antitrust scrutiny, after the enforcement agencies further pursue their studies.

On an even more immediate basis, government regulators (and potential prosecutors) have been following various means to reduce the perceived dominance of Blue Cross and Blue Shield by medical professionals. The FTC has expressed particular concern that where physicians dominate the insurer that reimburses for physician services, the insurer is unlikely to fulfill its functions of bargaining toward lower costs. Both the FTC and the Department of Health, Education and Welfare have pursued formal regulations to reduce this professional influence over the insurers, and the results could have an impact upon the separateness of providers and insurers, perhaps improving the viability of the current McCarran Act defense in ordinary situations, as the business of insurers (if not the "business of insurance") more clearly departs from the business of providers.

NOTES

1. 15 U.S.C. §§ 1011–1015.
2. 322 U.S. 533 (1944).
3. *See, Group Life and Health Ins. Co. v. Royal Drug Co.*, 99 S.Ct. 1067 (1979).
4. 90 Congressional Record A4405 (1944).

5. 91 Congressional Record 1481.

6. *See*, 90 Congressional Record A4406 (1944).

7. 15 U.S.C. § 1012.

8. 15 U.S.C. § 1013(b).

9. *Supra*, note 3.

10. *Id.*, at 4205.

11. *Id.*, at 4209.

12. *See, e.g., Frankford Hosp. v. Blue Cross*, 554 F.2d 1253 (3d Cir. 1977); *Anderson v. Medical Serv. of the District of Columbia*, 551 F.2d 304 (4th Cir. 1977).

13. 98 S.Ct. 2923 (1978).

14. 424 F. Supp. 657 (N.D. Cal. 1976); on appeal, the Ninth Circuit recognized that the trial court decision was inconsistent with the S.Ct.'s recent statement, and reversed, 1979–1 Trade Cases (CCH) ¶ 62,530 (1979).

15. *See, e.g., Travelers Ins. Co. v. Blue Cross*, 481 F.2d 80 (3d Cir. 1973); *Nankin Hosp. v. Michigan Hosp. Serv.*, 361 F.Supp. 1199 (E.D. Mich. 1973).

16. 518 F.2d 217 (5th Cir. 1975).

17. 556 F.2d 1375, 1385 (5th Cir. 1977).

18. *See*, Weller, "The McCarran-Ferguson Act's Antitrust Exemption For Insurance: Language, History and Policy" 1978 *Duke L.J.* No. 2, at 587–643.

19. *Id.*, at 617.

20. One notable exception to this conclusion is the approach of the court in *Allstate Ins. Co. v. Lanier*, 242 F. Supp. 73 (E.D. N.C. 1965), where a restrictive interpretation of state regulation was applied.

21. 15 U.S.C. § 1013(b).

22. *Supra*, note 13.

23. 557 F.2d 1001 (3d Cir. 1976).

24. 451 F. Supp. 624 (N.D. Va. 1978).

25. 543 F.2d 1075 (4th Cir. 1976); although this decision preceded *Barry*, it appears to conform entirely to the Supreme Court's later reasoning.

26. *See*, Antitrust and Trade Reg. Rep. (BNA) No. 897, Special Supplement, at 68.

Chapter 8

Price Discrimination: the Robinson-Patman Act

Price discrimination laws restrict sellers of *commodities* from charging "discriminatory" prices and sanction the knowing receipt by purchasers of favorable discriminations in price. Although health care providers are involved primarily in the delivery of *services,* they also are buyers and sellers of substantial amounts of commodities. A prime example—the subject of a major decision by the Supreme Court that is discussed in this chapter—is the purchase and resale of drugs and other pharmaceuticals by hospitals, either alone or, increasingly, through joint purchasing associations. Exposure to price discrimination liability, however, is not limited to this one area; hospitals also buy a variety of other commodities, from food to maintenance and building materials to hospital supplies, and equipment ranging from tongue depressors to CT scanners.

This chapter focuses on the most important of these laws, the federal antiprice discrimination statute known as the Robinson-Patman Act. As drafted by Congress and interpreted by the courts, the Robinson-Patman Act is anomalous. Its rules are so divergent from both general antitrust policy and economic notions of harmful price discrimination that it has been criticized as being inimical to competition. Critics say the primary effect of the act has been to stifle efforts by sellers to compete and by purchasers to negotiate for lower prices that in turn might be passed on to consumers. The act's defenders have contended that this is a reasonable trade-off to protect the viability of the small retailer from the "unfair" competition of chains and other more sizeable competitors that the defenders deem to be detrimental to society for reasons that are more political than economic.

To understand both how the Robinson-Patman Act works and why it sometimes has failed to work, a basic understanding of the economic definition of price discrimination is a prerequisite. Thus, before the act is analyzed in detail, a relatively nontechnical discussion of this topic follows.

THE ECONOMICS OF PRICE DISCRIMINATION

Price discrimination, as economists define it, occurs when an identical product is sold to different buyers at (1) different prices that are not justified by the difference in the relative costs of selling to those buyers, or (2) at the same price if the greater cost of selling to particular buyers is not accounted for by higher prices to those buyers.[1] Thus, price discrimination, in the economic sense, cannot be equated with price difference. It is not price discrimination to charge two customers different prices for a particular commodity if the disparity is based on the differing costs of producing and selling the commodity to those customers; in fact, to sell such a commodity to those two customers at the same price would constitute economic price discrimination. A different rate of return, where the difference is not based on cost and not on a different price, is the sign of economic price discrimination.[2]

Despite the pejorative connotations of the term, price discrimination, as economists view it, is not necessarily bad. In a competitive market, temporary economic price discrimination is an essential competitive tool, allowing sellers to test market responses[3] by, for example, selective price cutting. Long-run discrimination cannot exist if there is competition; the discriminating seller would be able to retain only his favored customers because his competitors soon would lure away the rest by charging them lower prices that accurately reflected the cost of production and sale.[4] One commentator has concluded:

> Persistent price differences in markets with rivals, therefore, are not price discriminations. They necessarily reflect differences in the cost of doing business with different customers. Such differences arise from a variety of factors, including the amounts customers purchase, selling costs, service costs, the performance of distributive functions by the customer, and so on. This fact means that the law should never attack price differentials of this sort.[5]

Thus, a price discrimination law that is effective in the economic sense should be aimed at the continuous form of price discrimination, which should not occur in a competitive market and therefore strongly indicates the existence of monopoly power.[6] However, as economists see it, the law should not attack the short-run discrimination that is characteristic of a competitive market or the breakup of a monopoly or cartel.[7]

THE NATURE OF THE ROBINSON-PATMAN ACT

The framers of the Robinson-Patman Act were lawyers and politicians rather than economists. Those who have used and interpreted the act over its life of more than four decades have been lawyers and judges. Thus, it is not surprising that the law of price discrimination owes little to economic theory and much to politics and the legal process.[8] The contrast between theory and practice is necessary to an understanding of the nature, development, and likely future of price discrimination law.

The Robinson-Patman Act[9] was passed by Congress in 1936 as a revision of Section 2 of the Clayton Act. The old Section 2 had been aimed at eliminating anticompetitive price cutting at the so-called "primary line," or among sellers, where the adverse impact was on the price cutter's direct competitors.[10] In addition to tightening the language of Section 2, which had been rendered virtually meaningless by court interpretation,[11] the Robinson-Patman Act added several new sections to deal with perceived abuses by large buyers, particularly retail chain stores.[12] Chain stores had been able to assert superior bargaining power to obtain price and price-related favorable discriminatory treatment from suppliers. These forms of discrimination included quantity discounts, advertising allowances, the charging of broker commissions without a broker's having been employed, and extra services performed by the suppliers.[13] Independent retailers, such as "mom and pop" grocery stores, complained that the chains (their direct competitors at the so-called "secondary line") were able to charge lower prices as a result of the unjustified concessions, making it impossible for the smaller buyers to compete effectively.[14]

Although not totally unrelated to economic theory, the legal definition of price discrimination in the Robinson-Patman Act could well be described as the illegitimate child of economic price discrimination theory. For example, it was noted earlier that a price difference did not necessarily constitute (and identical prices did not necessarily rule out) price discrimination. Nevertheless, "price discrimination" under the act has been consistently interpreted as synonymous with price difference.[15]

The act appears to take economics into account in providing a "cost justification" defense, allowing price "differentials which make only due allowance for differences in the cost of manufacture, sale, or delivery resulting from the differing methods or quantities" in which commodities are "sold or delivered."[16] In addition, the act allows a seller to defend "by showing that his lower price . . . *was made in good faith to meet an equally low price of a competitor* . . . ."[17] (emphasis added). However, these affirmative defenses have been criticized heavily as being at best virtually useless and at worst anticompetitive.[18] Although the seller may attempt to show that the price differentials were not discriminatory because they could be explained completely by cost differences, it is extremely difficult in practice to prove such cost justification effectively. The "meeting competition" defense allows the seller to escape liability only if the price differential is designed to "meet" his competitor's price; the defense generally has been unavailable to the seller who has engaged in good faith competition by beating his competitor's price.

Neither of these two defenses is designed to promote the kinds of price discrimination that economists view as beneficial to competition, and, indeed, the "meeting competition" defense has been viewed as having a perverse anticompetitive bias.[19] The effect of the act as a whole, and of the "meeting competition" defense in particular, has been characterized as being antithetical to the Sherman Act's price-fixing prohibition.[20]

Thus, it is not surprising that the act for many years has received what has been cumulatively described as "an avalanche of criticism" from all political viewpoints.[21] It also is not surprising that the act's major defender has been the interest group that was responsible for its passage initially: small businesses.[22] Despite considerable testimony favoring the act's repeal or substantial revision from members of Congress, the Justice Department, and the Federal Trade Commission, among others, no legislation emerged from the 1975 hearings by the House Small Business Committee's Ad Hoc Subcommittee on Antitrust, the Robinson-Patman Act, and Related Matters, largely because of the intense lobbying of small business associations.[23] Indeed, the Ad Hoc Subcommittee expressly recommended that no action be taken to "weaken, emasculate, or repeal the Robinson-Patman Act" and that the relevant Federal agencies "fully and effectively enforce the Robinson-Patman Act . . . to aid and assist the small business section of the American economy. . . ."[24] Because of the continued political strength of such associations, as well as some support in Congress and the legal community,[25] significant reform does not appear imminent. Although beleaguered, the act retains a substantial amount of vitality, and no business, including those in the health care industry, can afford to ignore it.

The act prohibits a seller from discriminating in price between different contemporaneous purchasers of commodities of like grade and quality where there is likely to be an anticompetitive effect, unless the discrimination is cost-justified or represents a good faith attempt to meet a competitor's price. This definition represents a summary of Sections 2(a) and (b), the key provisions of the act. Sections 2(c)-(e) prohibit certain brokerage payments and sellers' giving discriminatory payments and services to buyers. Most important from the standpoint of health care providers, which generally do not sell large quantities of commodities, is Section 2(f), which prohibits a buyer from knowingly inducing or receiving a discriminatory price.

Section 3 of the act, which is not an antitrust statute in the strict sense,[26] makes it a criminal offense for a seller to (1) grant secret rebates not offered to competing purchasers on goods of like grade, quality, and quantity, (2) engage in territorial price discrimination for the purpose of "destroying competition" or eliminating a competitor, or (3) charge "unreasonably low prices" for the same purpose, so-called "predatory pricing." That conduct also may violate Section 2(a) and Section 2 of the Sherman Act, and it probably is for this reason (as well as the absence of a private right of action) that there have been few cases under

Section 3.[27] Because of this overlap, and the relatively minor significance of Section 3, particularly insofar as health care providers are concerned, it will not be discussed further. The act's special jurisdictional prerequisites and its exemptions, the latter being particularly significant for nonprofit health care providers, are discussed below. The balance of the chapter analyzes the substantive provisions of the act,[28] with emphasis on Section 2(f), which has the most substantial impact on health care providers.

JURISDICTION

As noted in Chapter 1, "interstate commerce" is the threshold prerequisite for the application of the federal antitrust laws.[29] The concept of "commerce" is somewhat more technical and more limited under the Robinson-Patman Act (hereinafter "the act") than it is under the Sherman Act. The word "commerce" appears no fewer than four times in Section 2(a) (of the act):

> That it shall be unlawful for any person engaged in *commerce,* in the course of such *commerce* either directly or undirectly, to discriminate in price between different purchasers of commodities of like grade and quality, whether either or any of the purchases involved in such discrimination are in *commerce,* . . . and where the effect of such discrimination may be substantially to lessen competition or tend to create a monopoly in any line of *commerce.* . . .

The distinction between primary and secondary line competition once was thought to be of significance in determining whether the jurisdictional commerce requirement had been met. In 1954, the Supreme Court ruled in *Moore v. Mead's Fine Bread Co.* that in "primary line" cases where, for example, one drug manufacturer was alleged to have lessened competition substantially, to the injury of another drug manufacturer by selling at discriminatory prices (thus lessening competition in the primary line), the plaintiff needed only to prove that any of the defendant's sales crossed a state line.[30] In contrast, where a plaintiff distributor claims injury as a result of the defendant manufacturer's favorable discriminatory price to a competing distributor (thus lessening competition at the secondary line) the plaintiff could not satisfy the jurisdictional requirement unless it could be shown that the defendant made an interstate sale either to the plaintiff or to the rival.[31] However, it appears that the courts have eliminated this distinction, adopting the second rule in all cases, despite the fact that the *Moore v. Mead's Fine Bread Co.* "any sale" rule never has been expressly overruled.[32] Thus, it appears that the plaintiff must show in all Robinson-Patman Act cases that at least one of the defendant's discriminatory sales crossed a state line.[33] Based on the language of the act, the interstate transaction upon which jurisdiction is based must involve a commodity that is basically the same "grade and quality" as the commodity sold at a higher price intrastate, or the law is inapplicable.[34]

EXEMPTIONS

Although the jurisdictional requirements have been satisfied fully, a lawsuit under the act nevertheless may be dismissed if the allegedly discriminatory transactions fall within one of the following exemptions.

Nonprofit Organizations

For health care providers, the most significant of the Robinson-Patman Act exemptions is embodied in the Nonprofit Institutions Act of 1938 (also called the "Section 13c" exemption).[35] This exempts purchases of supplies for their own use by schools, colleges, universities, public libraries, churches, and, expressly, hospitals, and charitable institutions not operated for profit. In 1973, privately owned, nonprofit hospitals constituted 49 percent of all hospitals in the United States, representing 56 percent of nonfederal short-term hospitals and 70 percent of beds, or 80 percent of all nongovernmental hospitals.[36] The "charitable institutions" portion of the exemption similarly includes, in addition, all other nonprofit health care providers, including nonprofit intermediate care facilities and health maintenance organizations.

In March 1976, the Supreme Court ruled on the application of this exemption to direct purchases by hospitals and issued a set of uncharacteristically detailed and specific guidelines. In *Abbott Laboratories v. Portland Retail Druggists Association, Inc.,*[37] the court thus refused to exempt all of a nonprofit hospital's drug purchases from the act, but instead broke down the purchases into exempt and nonexempt categories, based on the types of people to whom they were sold or dispensed. The *Abbott* case arose when the Portland Retail Druggists Association brought an action under the Robinson-Patman Act as the legal representative of more than 60 commercial pharmacies in metropolitan Portland, Ore., charging that the 12 defendant manufacturers of pharmaceutical products discriminated against them in favor of nonprofit hospitals. The manufacturers contended in defense that the sales were exempt under the Nonprofit Institutions Act (hereinafter §13c).[38] The trial court ruled that almost all of the purchases were "for the use of the hospital" within the meaning of the Nonprofit Institutions Act, and that the number of resales by the hospital to walk-in patients was not of a sufficient magnitude to "justify withdrawing" the exemption.[39] The Court of Appeals for the Ninth Circuit vacated the trial court's decision, limiting the scope of the exemption to purchases destined for dispensation to hospital inpatients and emergency disability patients.[40]

The Supreme Court took a middle path, classifying the drug sales and dispensations into the following ten categories (using the court's numbering and language):

Exempt Sales

1. To the inpatient for use in his treatment at the hospital. For present purposes, we define an inpatient as one admitted to the hospital for at least overnight bed occupancy.
2. To the patient admitted to the hospital's emergency facility for use in the patient's treatment there. A patient in this category may or may not become an inpatient, as defined in the preceding paragraph.
3. To the outpatient for personal use on the hospital premises. For present purposes, we define an outpatient as one (other than an inpatient or a patient admitted to the emergency facility) who receives treatment or consultation on the premises.
4. To the inpatient, or to the emergency facility patient, upon his discharge and for his personal use away from the premises.
5. To the outpatient for personal use away from the premises.
7. To the hospital's employee or student for personal use or for the use of his dependent.[41]
8. To the physician who is a member of the hospital's staff, but who is not its employee, for personal use or for the use of his dependent.[42]

Non-Exempt Sales

6. To the former patient, by way of a renewal of a prescription given when he was an inpatient, an emergency facility patient, or an outpatient.
9. To the physician who is a member of the hospital's staff, for dispensation in the course of the physician's private practice away from the hospital.
10. To the walk-in customer who is not a patient of the hospital.[43]

The court's division between exempt and nonexempt purchases was based on what it called "the test . . . obvious [ly] . . . inherent in the language of the statute, namely, 'purchases of their supplies for their own use'. . . ."[44] The court then stated:

"[T]heir own use" is what reasonably may be regarded as use by the hospital in the sense that such use is *a part of and promotes the hospital's intended institutional operation in the care of persons who are its patients.*[45] (Emphasis added.)

Based on this test, the court excluded resales by former patients, stating that a prescription could not be for the hospital's " 'own use' forever simply because it originated under hospital auspices."[46] However, the court exempted take-home prescriptions, as follows:

[T]he genuine take-home prescription intended, for a limited and reasonable time, as a continuation of, or supplement to, the treatment that was administered at the hospital to the patient who needed, and now continues to need, that treatment, is for the hospital's "own use."[47]

Thus, the court resisted the temptation to draw a bright line test at the hospital's "doorsill."[48]

Next, purchases by the hospital's employee or its student were held to be exempt if they were for the buyer's or a dependent's own use, but not if they were for the use of another, "even a nondependent family member." The court rationalized this part of the rule:

A hospital is an organization populated by persons rendering essential services of various kinds. The hospital's employees enable it to function. The hospital pharmacy is but a part of the whole; the employee and his services are other parts. To the extent the institution has students on the medical and hospital scene . . . the connection with the hospital's purposes and its activities is obvious and institutionally intimate. We conclude, therefore, that dispensation by the pharmacy to the hospital's employee or student, each of whom, literally, is a member of the hospital family, for his own use or for the use of his dependent, enhances the hospital function and qualifies as being in the hospital's "own use" within the meaning of §13c.[49]

Although questionable from the standpoint of legal analysis, the inclusion of purchases for dependents is defensible as a judicial recognition of the impossibility of enforcing a rule exempting employees but not their dependents. However, some commentators have found it difficult to understand why hospital employees were included at all, arguing that if Congress had intended such a result the exemption would not have been limited to purchases for the hospital's "own use."[50]

Category nine states that sales to a physician "for dispensation in the course of the physician's private practice away from the hospital" are nonexempt.[51]

Elsewhere in the opinion, however, the court substitutes "unconnected with the hospital" for "away from the hospital."[52] This difference could be crucial, given the trend toward hospitals' leasing medical office space to nonemployee staff physicians, who have their own patients.[53] It could be argued that the prescriptions for these patients are not made "away from the hospital" and thus are exempt. The scope of category nine is far from certain, however, and probably will be the subject of future actions.

This interpretive problem also affects category three, where the court exempted sales made "to the outpatient for personal use on the hospital premises" and defined "outpatient" ambiguously as "one (other than an inpatient or a patient admitted to the emergency facility) who receives treatment or consultation on the premises."[54] This definition could include the physician's own patients, merely based on their having a "consultation" with the physician at his hospital-based office.[55]

Although category ten states that sales to walk-in customers are nonexempt, the court said later that "occasional" emergency walk-in dispensation cannot be the basis for a Robinson-Patman Act violation.[56]

Finally, the court considered the burdens its line-drawing rule would place on the hospital in requiring "a segregation of drugs or accounting of their use that can be achieved only through the institution of clumsy and expensive dual supplier tracing systems to regulate an account for the use of drugs."[57]

The court suggested two possible alternatives for the purchasing hospital. Under the first "and easier" alternative, the hospital's pharmacy would not make any nonexempt dispensations.[58] The potential financial and administrative hardships that would be attendant on such a sales limitation were completely ignored by the court. The second alternative would require the pharmacy to develop special accounting and recordkeeping procedures to segregate the exempt and nonexempt dispensations, "supplemented by the hospital's submission to its supplier of an appropriate accounting followed by the price adjustment that is indicated."[59] Anticipating critical response from hospitals and manufacturers, the court defended its position:

> This, to be sure, is cumbersome, but it obviously is the price that Congress has exacted for the benefits bestowed by the controlling legislation, and it should be no more cumbersome than the accounting demands that are made on commercial enterprises of all kinds in our complex society of today.[60]

Nevertheless, the difficulty and cost of complying with the *Abbott* decision has been criticized severely.[61] If these costs thus far have been less than might have been anticipated, this very likely is due to the fact that hospitals and other nonprofit institutions have eschewed strict compliance in favor of a *pro forma* version that pays mere lip service, both literally and figuratively, to the *Abbott* rule.[62]

There have been few other interpretations of the meaning of Section 13c. The only judicial interpretation prior to *Abbott* of the "own use" language under Section 13c was *Logan Lanes, Inc. v. Brunswick Corp.*[63] in 1967. In *Logan Lanes,* the Ninth Circuit liberally interpreted the "underlying intent" of Section 13c as being "undoubtedly to permit institutions which are not in business for a profit to operate as inexpensively as possible."[64] The Ninth Circuit then dismissed the action, which was based on discriminatory discounts in the sale of bowling lanes and equipment to a university's student union, based on the following "primary purpose test":

> The primary purpose of the purchases, established beyond dispute, was to fulfill the needs of the University in providing bowling facilities for its students, and staff. This being the case, any additional use of the bowling facilities by the general public for a fee, *even if such use is substantial, would not establish that the purchases were not made for the use of the University.*[65] (Emphasis added.)

In *Abbott,* the Ninth Circuit (which ruled on the case before the Supreme Court decision) had distinguished *Logan Lanes,* stating that, while it would be possible for a hospital to segregate drugs purchased for a hospital's "own use" from those bought for resale, "equipment acquired for a university's own use cannot be segregated from that acquired for use by others, since the same equipment serves both uses."[66] Thus, it appears that a nonprofit health care provider need not be concerned with accounting for nonexempt uses of equipment (as opposed to supplies) sold to it at a discount, although the Supreme Court in *Abbott* did not specifically address this portion of the Ninth Circuit's distinction.

The Federal Trade Commission in 1978 advised the Foundation for Later Life Enrichment, a nonprofit organization, that its plan to sell goods and services to the elderly at low prices would not qualify for the exemption because the goods involved would not be purchased for the institution's "own use."[67] Consequently, it is apparent that government enforcers are continuing to apply the nonprofit exemption in a limited manner. Good intentions or charitable motivations simply are not adequate in themselves to raise the defense.

Government Transactions

In 1974, 38 percent of the hospitals in the United States were federal, state, or local government institutions.[68] Although the Supreme Court has ruled that governmental agencies are not automatically exempt from the antitrust laws by reason of their status, and the statutory language is sufficiently broad to cover governmental bodies, it has been held that sales to the federal government or its agencies are exempt from the Robinson-Patman Act.[69] Federally owned hospitals, which in 1974 represented 5.5 percent of the nation's total but more than 9 percent of the average daily census of inpatients and more than 19 percent of outpatients,[70] thus are completely exempt from the act.

Sales to a state or municipality, or an agency thereof, generally have been held to fall within the same exemption.[71] An apparent exception is California, where the attorney general ruled in 1937 that the Robinson-Patman Act was applicable to government contracts but permitted price differentials based on quantity purchases, the absence of credit risks, solicitation expense, and other factors.[72] Another attorney general's opinion (Georgia's, in 1949) has held that a state acting in a proprietary capacity is subject to the act.[73] But the better rule appears to be that states and state agencies are exempt. A federal district court in 1978 concluded, after thorough analysis of case law and the legislative history of the act, that this exemption included state hospitals.[74] The court emphasized that the "state action" exemption (discussed in Chapter 3) is to be distinguished, as limited "to situations involving a 'state policy to displace competition with regulation or monopoly public services.' "[75] However, the "government transaction" exemption from the Robinson-Patman Act and the "state action" exemption from the antitrust laws could overlap if, for example, the state were to require all governmental purchases to be based on the lowest available price.

Cooperative Associations

Section 4 of the Robinson-Patman Act provides that a cooperative association is not prohibited from returning to its members all or any part of the net earnings or surplus resulting from its trading operations, in proportion to their purchases or sales from, to, or through the association.[76] The basic purpose of this provision is to protect and encourage cooperative buying and selling, with its positive competitive effects.[77] In *Mid-South Distributors v. FTC*,[78] the court held that Section 4 did not authorize cooperative associations to engage in practices prohibited by Section 2(f). Thus, cooperative buyers could not join together in a group for the purpose of receiving discriminatory prices from nonexempt sellers because the exemption protected a cooperative association only on charges growing out of the distribution of its earnings. Activities otherwise illegal under Section 2 of the Act are not protected.

Consequently, although the exemptions for governmental health care institutions and for nonprofit institutions (insofar as they are purchasing for their own use) protect a substantial percentage of health care institutions from Robinson-Patman Act liability, many still are subject to the act, at least with respect to some of their purchases and all of their sales of commodities. The act remains fully applicable not only to all discriminatory purchases by proprietary hospitals,[79] and other for-profit health care organizations such as proprietary Health Maintenance Organizations, but also to (1) the nonexempt discriminatory purchases and sales of nongovernmental, nonprofit health care institutions, and (2) all discriminatory sales and purchases by nonexempt entities owned or operated by, or affiliated with, or otherwise related to, any of these health care organizations. The next section of this chapter discusses how the act applies to such purchases.

BUYER LIABILITY FOR INDUCING OR RECEIVING DISCRIMINATORY PRICES

Section 2(f) of the Robinson-Patman Act makes it "unlawful for any person engaged in [interstate] commerce in the course of such commerce, . . . *knowingly to induce or receive* a discrimination in price. . . ."[80] (Emphasis added.) The jurisdictional elements are the same as under Section 2(a), as discussed earlier, except for the additional requirement that the defendant buyer must have been "engaged in commerce," and that the alleged discrimination must have occurred "in the course of such commerce."[81] After jurisdiction has been established and the relevant exemptions eliminated, two main elements must be proved to establish a buyer's violation under Section 2(f). First, the plaintiff must show that the buyer has received an unlawful price discrimination. Second, the plaintiff must show that the buyer had knowledge of the illegality.[82] Such knowledge is difficult to prove, but the FTC has been upheld by the courts in finding that "knowledge" for the purposes of Section 2(f) exists where: (1) the buyer pays a price that previously has been found to be illegal, (2) the buyer purchases in the same quantity and manner as any competitors, and (3) the buyer's experience in the trade should alert the individual to the lack of cost justification for the price difference.[83]

The affirmative defenses available to a seller also may be raised by a buyer defending under Section 2(f). The Supreme Court has stated:

. . . A buyer is not liable . . . if the lower prices he induces are either
(1) within one of the seller's defenses such as the cost justification or
(2) not known by him not to be within one of those defenses. . . .[84]

To rebut the buyer's assertion of the cost justification defense, the FTC need not prove lack of cost justification or good faith meeting of competition but only that the buyer knew or should have known that the discriminatory price was not so justified.[85] Thus the buyer must show that he or she did not know and could not reasonably have known of a flaw in the seller's purported affirmative defense. In one case, a chain grocer was found to have violated Section 2(f) by illegally accepting price concessions from a dairy, despite the dairy's having been absolved from liability based on the meeting competition defense.[86] In that case, the Court of Appeals for the Sixth Circuit concluded that the grocer knew that the low prices the dairy sought in good faith to meet had not in fact been offered by its competitor, but had induced the price concessions by representing the contrary to the dairy. Because of the buyer's deliberate misrepresentations, the grocer could not resort to the affirmative defense used by the seller, which was based on the latter's good faith ignorance.[87]

In a private Section 2(f) action, as opposed to one brought by the FTC, the plaintiff has the burden of establishing that the defendant knew or should have known that the lower prices were not cost justified or intended in good faith to meet competition.[88] Based on this rule, if the *Abbott* case had been brought against the purchasing hospitals under Section 2(f), rather than against the drug manufacturers under Section 2(a), the plaintiffs would have been required to prove that each hospital knew or should have known that the discounts it was receiving were not justified on the basis of either lower costs to the sellers or a good faith decision to meet competition. To defend successfully against such an action, the hospitals probably would need to show only that they knew they were purchasing greater quantities of drugs than the commercial pharmacies, and that the lower prices the hospitals paid thus appeared to be reasonable quantity discounts.[89]

Yet another obstacle to Section 2(f) actions is the general Robinson-Patman Act requirement that the plaintiff prove that the unlawful price discrimination had or is likely to have a substantial anticompetitive effect.[90] For example, the commercial pharmacies in *Abbott* would have had to show that they lost business to the hospital pharmacies because of the lower prices resulting from discriminatory discounts.[91] Although that issue was not decided in *Abbott,* arguably the only purchases that should be included in the determination of anticompetitive effect are those held to be nonexempt by the Supreme Court in that case. Such a requirement would compound the already substantial burden on Section 2(f) plaintiffs.

In light of these substantial obstacles to a successful private suit under Section 2(f), the chances of a successful treble damage action against a purchasing health care provider are reduced, despite recent increased use of Section 2(f).[92]

SELLER LIABILITY UNDER SECTIONS 2(a) AND (b)

Health care providers traditionally have not engaged in the kind of large-scale selling of commodities that may result in lawsuits against them under Sections 2(a) and 2(b) of the Robinson-Patman Act. However, providers are faced with an increasingly restrictive and even hostile regulatory environment, compounded

by the effects of ever-increasing inflation as well as intensified competition between fee-for-service providers and prepaid health service systems. Hospitals in
particular, because of their need for relatively large amounts of capital, will be
forced to find new ways of obtaining needed funds. One such method is investment in nonhealth-related companies, either by the hospital itself or through a
separate hospital foundation or other hospital-related entity. If a provider invests
in a firm that sells commodities interstate, the facility at least will be indirectly
within the potential scope of seller liability under Sections 2(a) and 2(b).

As noted previously, "price discrimination" in the meaning of Section 2(a)
has been held by the Supreme Court to mean "merely a price difference."[93]
However, quantity discounts, timely payment allowances, delivery services, and
the like may be considered in determining price, though usually such indirect
price discrimination is not the basis for an action under Section 2(a).[94] Section
2(e) deals expressly with discrimination in the providing of services, and thus
overlaps with the indirect price discrimination coverage of Section 2(a).[95]

A second requirement under Section 2(a) is that the seller has sold commodities of like grade and quality to at least two different purchasers. Leases and
other transactions lacking a "purchaser" are not covered.[96] In addition, the sales
must be reasonably contemporaneous.[97]

"Commodities" in the meaning of the act have been held not to include services or intangible "goods" such as advertising.[98] Thus, the kind of price discrimination that long has characterized the field of medicine,[99] which involves services, is beyond the scope of the act.

The commodities sold at discriminatory prices must be of "like grade and
quality." This requirement has been interpreted to mean "[a]ctual and genuine
physical differentiations between two different products adapted to the several
buyers' uses, *and not merely a decorative or fanciful feature. . . .*" (Emphasis
added.)[100] The Supreme Court has held that a difference in brand names does not
by itself mean that the two brands are not of "like grade and quality,"[101] though
this may be the result when the brands have physical differences that affect their
marketability.[102]

Finally, the plaintiff has the burden of proving that the price discrimination
has an anticompetitive effect, because it may (1) substantially lessen competition
or tend to create a monopoly in any line of commerce or (2) injure, destroy, or
prevent competition with any person who either (a) grants, or (b) knowingly
receives the benefit of such discrimination, or (c) with the customers of either of
them.[103] Part (1) of the above anticompetitive effects test is a part of the old
Clayton Act, Section 2, which was aimed at "primary line" injury to the seller's
competitors.[104] Part (2) is the Robinson-Patman Act's amendment to Section 2
of the Clayton Act and is aimed at "secondary line" injury to competitors of the
buyers.[105] Finally, the plaintiff must prove that the unlawful discrimination prox-
imately caused injury and measurable damages.[106]

The Cost Justification Defense

The cost justification defense was discussed briefly in the introduction to this chapter and again in the section on buyers' liability under Section 2(f). The burden of proving that the different prices charged to buyers merely takes into account the difference in cost between the two sales falls upon the defendant, as is the case with all of the defenses under Sections 2(a) and (b).[107] Defendants historically have encountered great difficulties in producing convincing evidence that prices for a particular customer were reduced because of cost savings based, for example, on lower production, delivery, or service costs. Cost accounts generally do not reflect the relative expense of selling to particular customers,[108] and it is rare that the defendant has such detailed accounting data available.[109] Although intangible cost savings based on accounting estimates have been allowed in some cases,[110] generally cost justification evidence must be "concrete and specific."[111] It is especially difficult to prove that the discrimination was justified by differences in the cost of manufacture because the Federal Trade Commission traditionally has allocated overhead on a uniform basis to all of the commodities sold.[112] The FTC has accepted a cost justification defense only where the reduced cost of manufacture can be tied directly to a specific purchaser, such as in the case of a special order.[113] As a result, the FTC rarely has accepted a cost justification defense, even where the defendant managed to justify a part of the discount that had been given; the Commission's order invariably has prohibited the seller from giving any discount, even to the extent justified.[114] Because of the high cost and apparent futility of attempting to prove cost justification, the defense is not used often.[115]

One analysis of the discriminatory sales in the *Abbott* case, discussed above in regard to the exemption for nonprofit institutions, concluded that the discrimination was difficult to explain but probably was based on the hospital's bargaining power.[116] If so, the cost justification defense would not be available. However, the reduced prices could be justified on the basis of lower seller costs based on the greater size of hospital pharmacy purchases, in comparison to those of commercial pharmacies. If such a defense is to succeed, however, drug manufacturers would have to produce detailed cost accounts documenting the savings in marketing, distribution, shipping or handling.

The Meeting Competition Defense

The other major defense, discussed in the introduction to this chapter and in the section on buyer liability, allows a seller to avoid Section 2(a) liability if the plaintiff's case can be rebutted by showing that the lower price "was made in good faith to meet the *equally low price* of a competitor. . . ."[117] (Emphasis added.) The "good faith meeting of competition" defense generally has been interpreted strictly, the usual rule being that the seller is entitled to match *but not beat*, the competitor's price.[118] The seller also must show that the price cut was made in good faith in response to a specific competitive situation.[119] If this latter test is satisfied, the seller in some situations may be allowed to beat the competitor's price if it is unrealistic to expect that price to be met precisely.[120] Once the elements of this defense have been established, it conclusively constitutes a complete defense to a charge of price discrimination, in spite of any anticompetitive effect that may result.[121]

In practice, however, this defense has been used rarely because of the difficulty of proving good faith and the general limitation of the defense to cases where the seller meets but does not undercut a competitor's price.[122]

Some commentators have noted that the application of the good faith meeting of competition defense to the health care industry is problematic, as a result of the mix of nonprofit and for-profit providers and thus of exempted and nonexempted transactions.[123] For example, where a proprietary provider expects a seller to meet a price offered to that proprietary's nonprofit competitor, problems may be encountered in establishing the meeting competition defense if the sale to the nonprofit institution was exempt initially from Robinson-Patman liability. The question may be resolved, however, by resorting to a factual analysis of the actual "good faith" of the parties and the actual "competition" between the institutions.

ILLEGAL BROKERAGE UNDER SECTION 2(c)

Under Section 2(c), brokerage commissions are unlawful *per se* unless made to an independent broker. The genesis of this section was explained by the Supreme Court,[124] as follows:

The Robinson-Patman Act was enacted in 1936 to curb and prohibit all devices by which large buyers gained discriminatory preferences over smaller ones by virtue of their greater purchasing power. A lengthy investigation revealed that large chain buyers were obtaining competitive advantages in several ways other than direct price concessions and were thus avoiding the impact of the Clayton Act. One of the favorite means of obtaining an indirect price concession was by setting up "dummy" brokers who were employed by the buyer and who, in many cases, rendered no services. The large buyers demanded that the seller pay "brokerage" to these fictitious brokers who then turned it over to their employer. This practice was one of the chief targets of § 2(c) of the Act. But it was not the only means by which the brokerage function was abused and Congress in its wisdom phrased § 2(c) broadly, not only to cover the other methods then in existence but all other means by which brokerage could be used to effect price discrimination.[125]

The court then went on to outlaw "split" brokerage, where the seller agrees to grant the buyer a lower price on the condition that the broker "split" or "share" part of the price cut by accepting a reduced brokerage commission.

Under Section 2(c), a plaintiff need not prove that any competitive injury resulted and the defendant may not escape liability by showing cost justification.[126] Despite the language of the section, which appears to provide an exception for payments "for services rendered," the defendant cannot escape Section 2(c) liability by showing that services actually were performed.[127]

Particularly significant from the perspective of health care providers is the fact that the law has been applied not only to mass distributors but also to brokerage collected by cooperative buying groups and passed on to the benefit of their members.[128] In one case, the brokerage held to be unlawful was collected by an agency created by 70 bakers to make cooperative purchases of supplies.[129]

Assuming that this rule retains its force, it will have to be considered by the increasing number of health care providers engaged in joint purchasing activity.

DISCRIMINATORY ALLOWANCES AND SERVICES UNDER SECTIONS 2(d) AND (e)

Sections 2(d) and (e) of the act, like Section 2(c), are intended to prohibit specific practices deemed to be anticompetitive in nature.[130] These provisions make it unlawful for the seller to give a buyer discounts for merchandising services rendered by the buyer to the seller (allowances), or for the seller to render such services to the buyer, unless they are made available to all buyers "on proportionally equal terms." To be "available" to all buyers under the act, the allowances or services need not actually be given or rendered to the buyers. However, they must be openly available to all buyers.[131] If the services offered cannot be used by some buyers, the seller must offer meaningful alternatives.[132]

A major issue under Sections 2(d) and (e) is the meaning of "on proportionally equal terms." The phrase could mean proportionality: (1) to the dollar volume of purchases made by various customers, or (2) to the cost to the buyer of the services rendered to the seller, or (3) to the value of such services to the seller. The FTC has adopted the first test, proportionality to dollar volume.[133]

As in Section 2(d), the plaintiff need not show anticompetitive effect and the defenses of cost justification and good faith meeting of competition are not available.[134] Services and allowances that are not provided "on proportionally equal terms" generally are illegal *per se*.[135]

OTHER PRICE DISCRIMINATION LAWS

At the federal level, discriminatory pricing and related practices also may be unlawful under Sections 1, 2, or 3 of the Sherman Act.[136] Many price discrimination cases are brought by the FTC because the broad language of Section 5 of the Federal Trade Commission Act has been held to cover varied kinds of discriminatory pricing and related practices that may be deemed unfair methods of competition or unfair practices.[137] Based on Section 5, the FTC has the power to attack as an unfair practice any activity contrary to the spirit of, but not expressly prohibited by, the Robinson-Patman Act.[138] Since the buyer has created the competitive situation that induced the discriminatory allowances, the FTC has taken the position that the good faith meeting of competition defense would not be available in such a case.[139] However, Section 4 of the Federal Trade Commission Act expressly excludes nonprofit entities from the purview of the FTC unless the entity is organized for the profit of its members.[140] As a result, for example, the American Medical Association and the American Hospital Association are covered by the act, but nonprofit hospitals and other nonprofit health care providers are outside the FTC's jurisdiction. In addition, associations composed entirely of nonprofit providers should be beyond the reach of the agency's enforcement powers.

Finally, a majority of the states have statutes prohibiting sales of commodities at prices that discriminate between different sections, communities, or cities.[141] Several of these statutes, such as those in Idaho, Oregon, Utah, Oklahoma, and Wisconsin, prohibit discrimination in the same area.[142]

NOTES

1. Areeda & Turner *Antitrust Law,* Vol. III (1978), at 186 (hereinafter Areeda & Turner); 186; Areeda, *Antitrust Analysis* (2d Ed. 1974), at 466 (Areeda). R. Bork, *The Antitrust Paradox* (1978), at 383 (Bork); R. Posner, *Antitrust Law* (1965), at 62 (Posner).

2. Bork, *id.,* at 388.

3. *Id.*

4. Areeda, *id.,* at 467.

5. Bork, *id.;* Adelman, "Book Review," 50 Amer. Econ. Ref. 790, 792 (1960).

6. Posner *id.,* at 63; Areeda, *id.,* at 467.

7. Posner, *id.*

8. For a thorough economic analysis, *see* J. Robinson, *The Economics of Imperfect Competition* (1933), ch. 15; Areeda, *id.,* at 466-468; Posner, *id.,* at 62-65, 178-180, 193-194, 242-243.

9. 15 U.S.C. § 13.

10. C. Wilcox, *Public Policies Toward Business* (4th ed. 1971), at 55 (hereinafter Wilcox).

11. *Id.,* at 200; *see Goodyear Tire and Rubber Co. v. FTC,* 101 F.2d (6th Cir. 1939) *cert. denied,* 308 U.S. 557.

12. *Id.,* at 55.

13. *Id.*

14. *Id.;* A.J. Rosoff & T. W. Dunfee, "A 'Fix' for the Retail Pharmacy: The Supreme Court Redefines Application of the Robinson-Patman Act to Drug Sales by Nonprofit Hospitals," 13 Cal. West. L. Rev. 195, 243 (1977); (hereinafter Rosoff & Dunfee) 1 Trade Reg. Rep. (CCH) ¶3200, at 5011.

15. F. Rowe, *Price Discrimination Under the Robinson-Patman Act* (1962, Supp. 1964) (hereinafter Rowe); Bork, at 383.

16. 15 U.S.C. § 13(a).

17. 15 U.S.C. § 13(b).

18. Rowe, at 534-55; *Department of Justice Report on The Robinson-Patman Act* (1977) (an outline of this report appears in 5 Trade Reg. Rep. (CCH) ¶ 50,311, at 55, 657 (1978)); Report of the Attorney General's National Committee to Study Antitrust Laws 191 (1955) (describing the act as "a legal quirk"); C. Edwards, *The Price Discrimination Laws* 624-27, 645-56 (1959); C. Kaysen & D. Turner, *Antitrust Policy: An Economic and Legal Analysis* 183-84 (1959); M. Green, *The Closed Enterprise System* 398-412 (1972); R. Posner, *The Robinson-Patman Act: Federal Regulation of Price Differences* (1976); "Justice Official Urges Robinson-Patman Repeal, Criticizes Act as 'Perverse,' Costly to Consumers," 737 Antitrust & Trade Reg. Rep. (BNA) A-6 (Nov. 4, 1975); Campbell & Emanuel, "A Proposal for a Revised Price Discrimination and Predatory Pricing Statute." 13 *Harv. J. L.* 125 (1975); F. Rowe, "The Robinson-Patman Act—Thirty Years Thereafter," 30 *ABA Antitrust Section* 9 (1966); Austern, "Isn't Thirty Years Enough?," 30 *ABA Antitrust* Section 18 (1966); Austern, "Difficult and Diffusive Decades: An Historical Plaint About the Robinson-Patman Act," 41 *N.Y.U. L. Rev.* 897 (1966); Steadman, "Twenty-Four Years of the Robinson-Patman Act," 1960 *Wis. L. Rev.* 197, 218 (describing the Act as "a hodge-podge of confusion and inconsistency that any competent, order-loving lawyer must find offensive").

19. *Id.;* Bork at 393-394.

20. Bork, at 394n; Levi, "The Robinson-Patman Act—Is It in the Public Interest?," 1 *ABA Antitrust Section* 60,61 (1952) (describing the act as "a price-fixing statute hiding in the clothes of antimonopoly and procompetition symbols.").

21. Rosoff & Dunfee, at 243; *see* note 18, *supra.*

22. *Id.,* at 244.

23. February 20, 1979, telephone conversation with a representative of the Small Business Committee of the United States House of Representatives.

24. 5 Trade Reg. Rep. (CCH) ¶ 50,289, at 55,597 (1978).

25. *See, e.g.,* E.W. Kintner, L.F. Henneberger, M.L. Fleischaker, "Reform of the Robinson-Patman Act: A Second Look," 21 *Antitrust Bull.* 203 (1976); B.J. Menzines, "The Robinson-Patman Act: A Current Appraisal," address by the executive director of the FTC before Automotive Warehouse Distributors Ass'n in Las Vegas, Nev., March 6, 1973, quoted in full in 5 Trade Reg. Rep. (CCH) ¶ 50,162, at 55,293.

26. *Nashville Milk Co. v. Carnation Co.,* 355 U.S. 373 (1958).

27. Areeda, at 866; *see, e.g., Moore v. Mead's Fine Bread Co.,* 348 U.S. 115 (1954) (involving both §§ 2 (a) and 3) and *United States v. National Dairy Prods. Corp.,* 372 U.S. 29, 37 (1963) (offering "unreasonably low prices" as sales below cost without legitimate commercial objective and with specific intent to destroy competition).

28. For a comprehensive analysis of the act, *see* F. Rowe, *Id.;* C. Edwards, *The Price Discrimination Law* (1969). Shorter analyses are provided in C. Austin, *Price Discrimination and Related Problems Under the Robinson-Patman Act* (2d ed. 1959) and K. Dam, "The Economics and Law of Price Discrimination: Herein of Three Regulatory Schemes, 31 *U.Chi.L.Rev.*1 (1963).

29. *See* jurisdictional considerations discussed generally in Ch.1.

30. *Moore v. Mead's Fine Bread Co.*, 348 U.S. 115 (1954).

31. *Mayer Paving and Asphalt Co. v. The General Dynamics Corp.*, 486 F.2d 763 (7th Cir., *cert. denied*, 94 S.Ct. 899 (1973); *Littlejohn v. Shell Oil Co.*, 483 F.2d 1140 (5th Cir., *cert. denied*, 94 S.Ct. 849 (1973). But compare *Gas-A-Car, Inc. v. Am. Petrofina, Inc.*, 484 F.2d 1102 (10th Cir. 1973).

32. *Willard Dairy Corp. v. Nat'l Dairy Products Corp.*, 309 F.2d 943 (6th Cir. 1962), *cert. denied* 373 U.S. 934 (1963); *Food Basket, Inc. v. Albertson's, Inc.*, 383 F.2d 785 (10th Cir. 1967). For a thorough treatment of this issue, *see* D. Salomon, "The Robinson-Patman Act Commerce Requirement: The Emasculation of Moore v. Mead's Fine Bread," 8 *U.S.F. L. Rev.* 497 (1974).

33. 1 Trade Reg. Rep. (CCH) ¶ 3270, at 5066 (1971).

34. *Central Ice Cream Co. v. Golden Rod Ice Cream Co.*, 287 F.2d 265 (7th Cir. 1961).

35. 15 U.S.C. § 13c (1970).

36. Cambridge Research Institute, *Trends Affecting the U.S. Health Care System* 296, 298 (DHEW 1975) (hereinafter DHEW Statistics).

37. 425 U.S. 1 (1976).

38. 425 U.S. at 4.

39. 425 U.S. at 7.

40. 425 U.S. at 8.

41. The court included "dispensation to a special duty nurse, chaplain, or similar nonemployee professional on duty at the hospital" in this category of exempt sales. 425 U.S. at 9, n.7.

42. 425 U.S. at 9-10.

43. *Id.*, the court observed that these ten categories "may not be exhaustive," but appeared "to cover, however, the several types of dispensations indicated by the record." 425 U.S. at 9-10, n.8.

44. 425 U.S. at 14.

45. *Id.*

46. 425 U.S. at 16.

47. 425 U.S. at 15.

48. *Id.*

49. 425 U.S. at 16.

50. Rosoff & Dunfee, at 215.

51. 425 U.S. at 10.

52. 425 U.S. at 17.

53. Rosoff & Dunfee at 213; Ludlam, "Physician-Hospital Relations: The Role of Staff Privileges," 35 L. & Contemp. Prob. 879, 882 (1970).

54. 425 U.S. at 9.

55. Rosoff & Dunfee, *id.*

56. 425 U.S. at 18.

57. Brief for Petitioners, p. 28, as quoted at 425 U.S. 20.

58. *Id.*

59. *Id.*

60. *Id.*

61. Rosoff & Dunfee, *id.*, at 217-230.

62. *Id.*, at 250-251. Such compliance consists largely of the pharmacy's sales clerks' asking customers whether they are patients, hospital employees, or employee dependents before ringing up the sale, with "nonexempt" persons being charged a few pennies more.

63. 378 F.2d 213 (9th Cir. 1967), *cert. denied*, 389 U.S. 989 (1967).

64. 378 F.2d 216.

65. 378 F.2d 217.

66. 510 F.2d 486, 490 (9th Cir. 1975)

67. 3 Trade Reg. Rptr. ¶ 21,457 (1979), at page 21,748.

68. DHEW Statistics, at 296.

69. *City of Lafayette v. Louisiana Power & Light Co.*, 437 U.S. 389 (1978) (governmental agencies not automatically exempt from antitrust laws); *but see Ops. Atty. Gen. of U.S.* (Dec. 28, 1932) 1932-39 Trade Cases (CCH) ¶ 55,0145, *General Shale Products Corp. v. Struck Const. Co.*, 37 F.Supp. 598 (D. Ky. 1941), *aff'd.* on other grounds 132 F.2d 425 (6th Cir. 1942) (sales to federal, state, or local governments not subject to Robinson-Patman Act).

70. DHEW Statistics, at 295; Rosoff & Dunfee, at 257, based on Table 3, *Hospital Statistics* 10-11 (1975).

71. *General Shale Products Corp. v. Struck Const. Co., supra,* note 69 *Jefferson County Pharmaceutical Ass'n, Inc. v. Abbott Laboratories,* Civ. No. 78-P-0807-S (N.D. Ala. Dec. 1, 1978); *Ops. Atty. Gen. of Minnesota,* (Mar. 4, 1937), 1932-1939 Trade Cases (CCH) ¶ 155,157. *But see, Ops. Atty. Gen. of California* (Feb. 26, 1937), 1932-1939 Trade Cases (CCH) ¶ 55,156.

72. *Opinion of Attorney General of California,* cited *supra,* note 71.

73. *Opinion of Attorney General of Georgia,* (June 14, 1949) 1948-1949 Trade Cases (CCH) ¶ 62,455.

74. *Jefferson County Pharmaceutical Association, Inc. v. Abbott Laboratories,* cited *supra,* note 71.

75. *Id.*

76. 15 U.S.C. § 15 (1970).

77. 1 Trade Reg. Rep. (CCH) ¶ 3280, at 5071.

78. 287 F. 2d 512 (5th Cir. 1961); *See also, Am. Motors Specialties Co. v. FTC,* 278 F.2d 255 (2d Cir. 1960).

79. DHEW Statistics, at 296, 299, indicates that in 1974 proprietaries represented approximately 12 percent of all U.S. hospitals.

80. 15 U.S.C. § 13(f).

81. *Mid-South Distributors v. FTC,* 287 F.2d 512 (5th Cir. 1960), *cert. denied,* 368 U.S. 838 (1961); *Am. Motor Specialties Co. v. FTC,* 278 F.2d 225 (2d Cir. 1960).

82. Practising L. Inst. *18th Annual Antitrust Law Institute* 261 (1977).

83. *Automatic Canteen Co., Inc. v. FTC,* 346 U.S. 61 (1953).

84. *Id.*

85. *The Great Atlantic & Pacific Tea Co., Inc.* Trade Reg. Rep. (CCH) ¶ 21,150 (FTC 1976); *Kroger Co. v. FTC,* 438 F.2d 1372 (6th Cir. 1971), *cert. denied,* 404 U.S. 871.

86. *Kroger Co. v. FTC,* cited *supra,* at note 85.

87. Compare *Great Atlantic and Pacific Tea Co., Inc. v. FTC,* 1979-1 Trade Cases (CCH) ¶ 62,475 (U.S. Supreme Court February 22, 1979), which did not involve such a "lying buyer" situation, because the seller's offer had been beaten by a competitor's first offer, and thus resulted in a decision in favor of the defendant buyer. The Supreme Court left open the question of whether even a lying

buyer would be liable under Section 2(f) if the seller has a meeting competition defense, as the Sixth Circuit had held in *Kroger*, cited *supra* at note 85.

88. *Automatic Canteen Co., Inc. v. FTC*, cited *supra* at note 83; *Holleb & Co. v. Produce Terminal Cold Storage Co.*, 532 F.2d 29 (7th Cir. 1976); *Texas Gulf Sulphur Co. v. J.R. Simplot Co.*, 418 F.2d 793 (5th Cir. 1959).

89. Rosoff & Dunfee at 251.

90. *American Motors Specialties Co., Inc. v. FTC*, cited *supra*, note 81; *FTC v. Sun Oil Co.*, 371 U.S. 505 (1963); *Borden Co. v. FTC*, 381 F.2d 175 (5th Cir. 1967); *Am. Oil Co. v. FTC*, 325 F.2d 101 (7th Cir. 1963); *cert. denied*, 377 U.S. 954 (1964); *Whitaker Cable Corp. v. FTC*, 239 F.2d (7th Cir. 1956), *cert. denied*, 353 U.S. 938 (1957).

91. Rosoff & Dunfee, at 253, where the authors also point out, at note 245, that the plaintiffs would have great difficulty proving anticompetitive impact unless the hospitals were able to provide "appropriately segregated data of their past sales," which the authors interpret to mean data that would enable the plaintiffs to trace usage according to the Supreme Court's categories of exempt and non-exempt transactions. They note that "[t]here is considerable doubt whether many hospitals currently maintain records of [this] sort."

92. Rosoff & Dunfee, at 253; Comment, "Buyer Liability for Inducing or Receiving Discriminatory Prices, Terms, and Promotional Allowances: Caveat Emptor in the 1970s," 7 *Ind. L. Rev.* 962 (1974).

93. *FTC v. Anheuser-Busch, Inc.*, 363 U.S. 536, 549 (1960).

94. *Guyott Co. v. Texaco, Inc.*, 261 F.Supp. 942 (D. Conn. 1956); *Clausen & Sons, Inc. v. Theo. Hamm Brewing Co.*, 284 F.Supp. 148 (D. Minn. 1967), *rev'd on other grounds*, 395 F.2d 388 (8th Cir. 1968).

95. Areeda, at 845 n.10, noting that discriminatory credit terms were held in *Clausen & Sons* to be covered under § 2(a) but not § 2(e), which was interpreted as dealing only with promotional services or facilities.

96. *Loren Specialty Mfg. Co. v. Clark Mfg. Co.*, 241 F.Supp. 493 (N.D. Ill. 1965), *aff'd*, through 60 F.2d 913 (7th Cir. 1966), *cert. denied*, 385 U.S. 957 (1966) (transaction that involved an agent was not covered).

97. Compare *Atalanta Trading Corp. v. FTC*, 258 F.2d 365 (2d Cir. 1958) with *Fred Meyer, Inc. v. FTC*, 359 F.2d 351 (9th Cir. 1966); *Joseph A. Kaplan & Sons v. FTC*, 347 F.2d 785 (D.C. Cir. 1965).

98. *Baum v. Investors Diversified Serv., Inc.*, 409 F.2d 872 (7th Cir. 1969); *Tri-State Broadcasting Co. v. United Press International, Inc.*, 369 F.2d 268 (5th Cir. 1966); Rowe, at 59-62.

99. *See generally* R. Kessel, "Price Discrimination in Medicine," 1 *J. of L. and Econ.* 20 (1958).

100. *Report of the Attorney General's Nat'l Comm. to Study the Antitrust Laws* 158 (1955).

101. *FTC v. Borden Co.*, 383 US637, 645-646 (1966).

102. *Universal-Rundle Corp.*, 65 FTC 924, 955 (1964), *set aside on other grounds*, 352 F.2d 831 (7th Cir. 1965), *rev'd* 387 U.S. 244 (1967).

103. Areeda, at 846; 1 Trade Reg. Rep. (CCH) ¶ 305, at 5089.

104. The leading Supreme Court case on "primary line" injury is *Utah Pie Co. v. Continental Baking Co.*, 386 U.S. 685 (1967). This decision has received particularly harsh criticism as being itself anticompetitive. *See, e.g.*, Bork, at 386-387; Bowman, "Restraint of Trade by the Supreme Court: The *Utah Pie* case," 77 *Yale L.J.* 70 (1967).

105. The leading Supreme Court case on "secondary line" injury is *FTC v. Morton Salt Co.*, 334 U.S. 37 (1948), which also has been severely criticized for its view that any price differential is likely to threaten injury to competition. Bork, at 391. Other leading cases on "secondary line"

injury include *American Oil Co. v. FTC*, 325 F.2d 101 (7th Cir. 1951), *cert. denied*, 344 U.S. 206 (1952). *See also, Report of Attorney General's Nat'l Comm. to Study the Antitrust Laws 207-208 (1955).*

106. *Fowler Mfg. Co. v. Gorlick*, 415 F.2d 1248 (9th Cir. 1959), *cert. denied*, 396 U.S. 1012 (1970); *Enterprise Industries, Inc. v. Texas Co.*, 240 F.2d 457 (2d Cir. 1957) *cert. denied*, 353 U.S. 965 (1957); *Krieger v. Texaco, Inc.*, 373 F. Supp. 108 (W.D.N.Y. 1953).

107. *Nagler v. Admiral Corp.*, 248 F.2d 319 (2d Cir. 1957); *FTC v. Morton Salt Co.*, 334 U.S. 37 (1948).

108. Wilcox, at 209.

109. *Id.*

110. *See, e.g., Reid v. Harper & Bros.*, 235 F.2d 420 (2d Cir. 1956).

111. 1 Trade Reg. Rep. (CCH) ¶ 3350, at 5213.

112. Wilcox, at 210.

113. Rosoff & Dunfee, at 254, citing E. W. Kintner, *A Robinson-Patman Primer*, (1970), at 174.

114. Wilcox, *Id.*

115. *Id.*

116. Rosoff & Dunfee, at 255-256.

117. 15 U.S.C. § 13(b).

118. *Moss, Inc. v. FTC*, 148 F.2d 378 (2d Cir. 1945), *cert. denied*, 326 U.S. 734 (1945).

119. *FTC v. A.E. Staley*, 324 U.S. 746 (1945).

120. *Kroger Co. v. FTC*, cited *supra*, note 85.

121. *Standard Oil Co. v. FTC*, 340 U.S. 231 (1951).

122. Wilcox, at 211-212.

123. *See, e.g.*, Rosoff & Dunfee, at 256-257.

124. *F.T.C. v. Henry Broch & Co.*, 363 U.S. 166 (1960).

125. 363 U.S. 168-169.

126. *Biddle Purchasing Co. v. FTC*, 96 F.2d 687 (2d Cir. 1938), *cert. denied*, 305 U.S. 634 (1938).

127. *A & P v. FTC*, 106 F.2d 667 (1939), *cert. denied.* 308 U.S. 625 (1940).

128. *Biddle Purchasing Co. v. FTC*, cited *supra*, note 126.

129. *Quality Bakers v. FTC*, 114 F.2d 393 (1st Cir. 1940).

130. Areeda, at 928.

131. Wilcox, at 203-204.

132. Wilcox, at 203.

133. Wilcox, at 204.

134. Areeda, at 928; *FTC v. Simplicity Pattern Co.*, 360 U.S. 55 (1959).

135. *Vanity Fair Paper Mills, Inc. v. FTC*, 311 F.2d 480 (2d Cir. 1962); *FTC v. Fred Meyer, Inc.*, 390 U.S. 341 (1968).

136. 1 Trade Reg. Rep. (CCH) ¶ 3460, at 5370.

137. *Id.*, ¶ 3470, at 5379; *Grand Union Co. v. FTC*, 300 F.2d 92 (2d Cir. 1962); *see generally*, 1 Trade Reg. Rep. (CCH) ¶¶ 800 *et seq*, at 1601.

138. *Fred Meyer, Inc. v. FTC*, 359 F.2d 351 (9th Cir. 1966), *reversed on other grounds*, 390 U.S. 341. For example, the FTC may enjoin a buyer from inducing or receiving discriminatory allowances, and need not establish injury to competition. 1 Trade Reg. Rep (CCH) ¶ 3470, at 5381.

139. *Max Factor & Co.*, Dkt. 7717, discussed at 1 Trade Reg. Rep. (CCH) ¶ 3470 at 5380-5381.

140. 15 U.S.C. § 44.
141. 1 Trade Reg. Rep. (CCH) ¶ 3510, at 5401.
142. *Id.*

Chapter 9

Particular Considerations for Directors and Trustees

As discussed previously, hospitals and other health care providers must walk a thin line between complying with voluntary and compulsory measures designed to control costs and engaging in such extensive cooperation with their competitors, even in the name of cost containment, that they may be subject to legal sanctions for anticompetitive conduct. This chapter will discuss instances where such behavior can lead to individual liability of the directors or trustees of the provider corporation and will outline the steps ordinarily available to prevent such individual liability.

CORPORATE INTERLOCKS AND INDIVIDUAL LIABILITY

Anticompetitive conduct by a corporation may constitute a violation of federal or state antitrust statutes and lead to civil or criminal liability. The federal and state governments can bring antitrust suits, either civil or criminal, and may include directors as defendants. Suit also may be brought by a private party against the corporation, and treble damages sought for the antitrust violation.[1] An action may be brought directly against the directors (or some of them), in appropriate circumstances, and a corporation may seek indemnification from directors after a judgment against the corporation, especially if their action was not undertaken in good faith.[2] Recent amendments to federal law also permit state attorneys general to sue in the name of citizens injured, in their capacity as consumers, by violations of the antitrust laws.[3]

Interlocking Directorates

Similarly, the personal and independent activities of directors and trustees can lead to antitrust ramifications based upon a finding of interlocking directorates in violation of federal law.[4] Section 8 of the Clayton Act provides in substance that no person may, at the same time, act as a director in two or more competing corporations engaged in commerce, any one of which has certain assets exceeding $1 million.[5] "Competing corporations" are defined as those whose business and location are such that the elimination of competition by agreement between them would constitute a violation of any antitrust law.

The evils of corporate interlocks have been decried for at least a century. The problem, it seems, is to prevent direct competitors[6] from sharing directors and thus information of competitive value. It has long been felt, if never proved, that a director serving on the boards of competing companies would report price and other competitive information back to his principal company, if not back and forth, and adversely affect competition in the industry. Similarly, even if no price fixing arose as a result of such a relationship, it would facilitate the creation of informal noncompetition agreements, market division, and so forth. It has been argued that even indirect interlocks—those arising where two competing firms each have a director on the board of a third or, conversely, where a third corporation has directors on the boards of both competing corporations, threaten these evils.[7]

Section 8 applies only to competing corporations engaged "in commerce," thus reaching those that do business in more than one state as, for example, by making interstate purchases or sales. In addition, the federal legal requirements come into play only for corporations with "capital, surplus, and undivided profits" aggregating more than $1 million. Despite the presence of the term, "profits," there is no assurance that nonprofit health care providers would escape these provisions, since their capital may readily exceed the required $1 million and "profits" might be defined to equal "net revenues." In any case, large proprietary institutions or chains would be subject to these directives. Smaller institutions, even if outside the federal purview,[8] could be cited under state laws if it were argued successfully that similar arrangements were not in good faith, or not in the best interest of the corporation, or otherwise a violation of state law.

If the corporations are "in commerce" and at least one of them meets the minimum size requirement, a violation of Section 8 is established simply on a showing that the corporations are competitors so that the elimination of competition by agreement between them would constitute a violation of the antitrust laws. There is no requirement of showing that the dual directorship has the effect, or even the potential, of restraining competition.[9]

Note that no agreement (e.g., fixing prices or dividing markets) nor even the likelihood of such an agreement need be shown.[10] It is sufficient to show that were there an agreement to eliminate competition, the antitrust laws would be violated. And the fact that the volume of competing business was small compared to the corporations' total sales, or to the total volume of all sales of such items, does not vitiate the unlawfulness of the interlock.[11] In short, interlocking directorates among competitors of the required size are *per se* forbidden.

Section 8 of the Clayton Act may be enforced by either the Justice Department or the Federal Trade Commission,[12] which may seek injunctive relief against both the corporation and the common director.[13] There also has been at least one shareholders' derivative action seeking to end interlocking directorships that allegedly contravened Section 8.[14] In addition, cases brought by competitors on occasion have included Section 8 charges.[15] In any such claim, the director most likely would have a choice as to which position to resign; however, this is unclear because both enforcement and civil actions customarily are dismissed once the interlocking directorship has been discontinued.[16] Despite the apparent ease of resolving Section 8 difficulties, the more prudent course for both director and corporation is to avoid interlocks whenever possible.

Liability at Common Law

Directors' liability is possible for violation of the antitrust statutes, as seen. Anticompetitive conduct also might be argued to be a violation of a director's duties to the institution. The general standards of conduct for directors are well known: they must discharge their duties in good faith, acting in what they believe to be the corporation's best interest, and exercising the care an ordinarily prudent person would in like circumstances.[17] In doing so, they may rely on information and opinions from reliable employees and outside professionals.[18] This statutory mandate is close to the common law requirement of the exercise of reasonable care by a prudent person.

Most attention in this connection is focused on such areas as personal conflicts of interest and self-dealing, along with securities law violations and, recently, illegal payments and distributions. All of these are important, and many may affect directors of hospitals and other health care providers. None arise particularly out of antitrust regulation. Bearing classic antitrust inquiries in mind, however, it is possible to foresee situations where directors may be exposed to liability for the consequences of anticompetitive decisions.

Thus, if a hospital director is a member of the boards of two competitive institutions where the two directorates interlock impermissibly, and the interlock leads to antitrust liability on the part of the corporation, that director might be held to have violated the duty of care.[19] A similar violation might be found if the institution took action— negotiated a merger,[20] made purchases, entered into contracts such as nonduplication agreements or supply agreements—that might be held to interfere with competition.

Many types of activities by a health care provider might lead to antitrust claims against the directors as well as the institution itself. Generally, however, major institutional decisions that require the actual consideration and approval of the trustees or directors, such as mergers, acquisitions, and expansion programs, are the areas likely to lead to actions against those individuals. Areas of activity in which directors have personal stakes and therefore may be acting in their individual capacities, as well as their institutional ones, also are apt to attract antitrust attention.

Another, more roundabout approach to antitrust violations by debt or equity holders in the institution could be taken through federal (where applicable) and state securities laws. To the extent that a health care provider corporation is required to comply with securities law disclosure requirements, and to the further extent that pending or impending litigation (*e.g.*, antitrust litigation) must be disclosed under those requirements, directors could incur liability under state and/or federal disclosure statutes for failing to disclose antitrust violations.[21]

Direct or Secondary Liability

In each of the cited examples, the director's liability could be secondary. That is, only after the corporation was adjudged guilty of an antitrust violation would the director's liability to indemnify the corporation arise.

That liability could be direct, however, if the director was an active participant in the antitrust violation.[22] Under federal law, liability also is direct when directors order or authorize the illegal acts. The Clayton Act makes directors of corporations that violate its penal provisions guilty of a misdemeanor if they authorized, ordered, or did any of the acts.[23] In the language of the Clayton Act, "such violation shall be deemed to be also that of the individual directors . . . who shall have authorized, ordered or done any of the acts constituting in whole or in part such violations. . . ."[24] Thus, it can be important for directors to register their dissenting votes to activities they believe to be questionable.[25] Indeed, at least one federal court has held that the failure of a corporate director to take positive steps to correct an illegal corporate action was equivalent to active participation in it.[26] The failure of a corporate director to comply in good faith with an order to end an antitrust violation would subject the director to additional liability.

TYPES OF LIABILITY

Trustees and directors can incur a number of different kinds of liability. They may be held liable to third persons suing them directly; to shareholders or members suing them directly; or to the corporation, either in a suit by the corporation against them, or in a derivative action brought by one or more shareholders on behalf of the corporation. Finally, they may be liable civilly or criminally to a government entity bringing an action against them or against the corporation on whose board they serve. Essentially, the same facts could give rise to any of these claims, with the differences being in parties to the action and, possibly, the consequences to the director.

Direct Suits

Suits by third persons for antitrust violations are probably the greatest risk faced by directors. For example, one provider might sue another for its misconduct in opposing a certificate of need application. The applicant might contend that the opposition of the other provider was based on a desire to monopolize the service it offered and that the second facility sought to add, or on a desire to prevent the applicant from offering a service the opponent did not offer. Either way, the motives of the opponent would be characterized as anticompetitive, rather than based on a sincere interest in cost containment.[27]

A highly publicized case that may exemplify the appropriate concern of officers as well as directors and trustees of health care providers is *Hospital Building Co. v. Trustees of Rex Hospital.*[28] In *Rex,* a hospital administrator and a hospital trustee were alleged to have acted in concert with an official of a local health planning agency to block the relocation of a competing hospital operated by the plaintiff. The defendants contended that even if the plaintiff's allegations were proved, their 49-bed local hospital had an insufficient effect on interstate commerce to meet the jurisdictional requirement of the federal statute. The Supreme Court disagreed, holding that a sufficient impact on interstate commerce was shown, and the case was sent back for trial. Consequently, a cause of action was stated against officers and directors in their personal capacities.

Corporate directors also are subject to criminal prosecution where antitrust violations amount to criminal conduct. In *United States v. Wise,*[29] the Supreme Court held that the section of the Sherman Act imposing criminal sanctions on "every person" knowingly participating in an illegal combination in restraint of trade[30] subjected a corporate officer to prosecution whether he authorized, ordered or merely aided the illegal action.[31] Although the decision dealt with corporate officers, the reasoning of the court[32] would be equally applicable to directors and, where appropriate, to trustees.

Derivative Actions

The concepts of direct suit by third parties or of governmental actions against corporate directors mentioned above are relatively familiar. However, a word must be said about an additional, perhaps less familiar, type of suit a director can encounter: the derivative action. In such an action, a shareholder[33] brings suit against directors or other corporate wrongdoers and against the corporation itself. Although the suit is brought by the shareholder, courts have held that that individual is "a mere nominal plaintiff" and that "the corporation is the real party in interest, and any judgment recovered inures to its benefit."[34]

The derivative action permits shareholders to enforce rights belonging to the corporation when the corporation itself declines to do so.[35] It has long been held that shareholders may not sue on their own behalf for a wrong done to the corporation even if such a wrong reduced the value of their stock.[36] The availability of the derivative action assures the shareholder a mechanism for self-protection. While derivative actions generally are brought to obtain money recoveries, shareholders also may use the device to enjoin illegal action such as a proposed merger. Thus, where a shareholder had notice of proposed corporate action that threatened an antitrust violation, a derivative suit might be used to prevent the action from being taken at all.[37]

Originally an invention of the equity courts, derivative actions today are governed by state statutes. Although the statutes vary, there are three conditions generally imposed: (1) the plaintiff shareholder must have owned shares in the corporation at the time of the alleged wrong—the so-called "contemporaneous ownership" requirement; (2) the shareholder must have made a demand on the board of directors to act, or otherwise exhausted intracorporate remedies, unless such action would have been futile; and (3) if the court so orders, the plaintiff shareholder must post security for the expenses of litigation.[38]

Although the requirement of security for expenses has been seen as something of a deterrent to derivative actions, there have been some statutory revisions to diminish this deterrent effect[39] and in any case the derivative action remains as a very real enforcement tool in many situations. Nonetheless, its existence does not mean a board must sue whenever requested by a shareholder to do so. Indeed, some courts have held that where a board of directors acting by an independent majority not implicated in the alleged wrongdoing decides not to bring suit, the shareholder will be precluded from bringing a derivative action.[40]

If a derivative action is filed against them, the directors nonetheless may wish to reconsider prosecution of the action by the corporation. This can be done by filing a cross-complaint asserting the same claims against the remaining defendants. This action is permitted because in a derivative action, the plaintiff shareholder serves simply to set the court's judicial machinery in motion.[41] Indeed, since the goal is to vindicate a right of the corporation, the move should be seen as desirable and, where undertaken in good faith, will not be appealable by the original plaintiff, who will have become a supernumerary party.[42]

If the corporation does not choose to to become an active plaintiff in a derivative suit, it may not defend the action as a corporation since, if the plaintiff is successful, the company will be the beneficiary of any monetary recovery. Some statutes do permit a corporation to advance money to the other defendants to cover their expenses of litigation if they agree to reimbursement should it later be determined that they are not entitled to that financial help.[43] However, it would be improper for the corporation to pay the defendants' legal expenses to any greater extent.[44] Although some courts have held that the same counsel may represent both the corporation and the individual director defendants,[45] such dual representation might be ethically questionable.[46]

PROTECTING THE CORPORATE DIRECTOR

The threat of personal liability for conduct as a trustee or director has caused some observers to conclude that it will become more and more difficult to fill directorships with qualified persons.[47] This possibility has been further exacerbated by the public's changing perception of corporation directorship: what once was an honorable sinecure has been tainted by revelations of improper payments, illegal contracts, and other unsavory practices, and has become a time-consuming enterprise. The number of cases imposing liability on directors—and the even larger number in which such liability is sought—may give prospective directors serious pause. These cases, and recent regulatory moves, also indicate that more stringent requirements, making greater demands on directors' time and energy, will become the rule. At the same time, an emphasis on avoiding corporate interlocks[48] will increase the number of directors needed, as corporations seek only persons not serving on boards of other corporations, to help avoid antitrust difficulties.

Hospitals and other institutional providers, like other corporations, now face these multiple difficulties. They may well have directors who serve on the boards of financial institutions or insurance companies with which they deal. They may have community leaders on their boards who also are on the boards of other health care providers in the community. Or a local business leader, who happens to be in the pharmaceutical, hospital supply, or laundry business, or who may control a corporation that is a major purchaser of health care services from local providers, may serve as one of many board members.

Such direct and indirect interrelationships should receive careful scrutiny from management and counsel to ensure that both the institution and the directors comply with legal requirements. Even where technical legal requirements are not violated, the institutions and individuals involved may well consider areas of actual or apparent conflict or impropriety that may occur from joint control or direction of entities involved in otherwise independent business relationships.

Preventive Action

One basic but often elusive way to protect directors from such liability is to avoid foreseeable violations or questionable conduct. Management and counsel should evaluate areas where potential antitrust problems exist and govern the corporation in such a way as to avoid them. Antitrust and other litigation is not likely to be in the corporation's best interest, and it is important that directors and management be aware of likely problems and act to avoid them. Antitrust counseling thus might be a component part of the internal audit procedures pursued by providers, as well as other institutions, given the present atmosphere of concern with proper corporate governance.[49] Such counseling is particularly important in view of cases such as *United States v. Charles Pfizer & Co.*, where it was held that the mere belief by the corporate officials that conduct was lawful did not preclude their liability for such conduct.[50]

Such counseling likewise should be a part of the orientation given new board members.[51] It is necessary to impress directors, both inside and outside,[52] with the importance of their task and the need for them to spend the time and effort necessary to reasonably evaluate decisions they make on behalf of the corporation. The concern with avoiding corporate interlocks should facilitate such concentration because where fewer directorships are appropriate for any individual, each person should have more time to spend on behalf of a given board.

In addition, it is essential to recall that directors do not incur absolute liability for their actions, nor do they become insurers for the corporations they serve. Their conduct will be tested by the standards of reasonable care and business judgment, and they will be required only to act as reasonably prudent persons in like circumstances.[53]

In summary, to the extent the answer to a given dilemma is unclear, a director should not incur liability if the individual makes a reasonable choice. Of course, it would be preferable to avoid questionable conduct raising potential antitrust issues entirely rather than to avoid liability only after litigation. It is even more vital, however, to assure directors and trustees that they may exercise their reasonable business judgment in an unfettered fashion. This goal, always desirable, will become even more so in view of the creativity that will be necessary to meet both the requirements in this field and such apparently contradictory ones as those in the cost containment area.

Finally, to the extent permitted by statute and by corporate charters and bylaws, insurance may be provided to protect directors from liability for their good faith decisions and to protect the provider, as well, from any duty to indemnify directors from its own funds.

Indemnification and Insurance

The extent to which a corporation may indemnify a director for expenses incurred in connection with claims arising out of the person's official conduct is defined statutorily in most states. Generally, a director may be indemnified for liability resulting from a civil action by a shareholder or a third person or resulting from a criminal or administrative proceeding if the individual acted in good faith and in what the person reasonably believed to be the best interest of the corporation, without reasonable cause to believe that the conduct was unlawful.[54] There is no requirement of a favorable termination of the proceeding—only of a good faith belief. Indemnification includes expenses, judgments, fines, and settlements actually and reasonably incurred.

In shareholders' derivative proceedings and those brought by the corporation, the company may indemnify a director for expenses actually and reasonably incurred to defend claims arising out of the performance of the individual's corporate functions if the director acted in good faith.[55] Indemnification is directed by statute for actual and reasonable expenses in derivative and in third-party suits where the director is successful on the merits.[56] Where the result is adverse to the director, indemnification is permitted only to the extent the court finds it appropriate.[57] No indemnification is permitted for amounts paid in settlement or expenses incurred in connection with the legal action.[58] In any other case, indemnification is proper only when not prohibited by the corporate articles and bylaws and where authorized by a majority vote of disinterested directors or shareholders, or by the court itself.[59]

The corporation, however, may advance funds for expenses prior to judgment so long as the director agrees to repay the money unless the individual is found to be entitled to indemnification.[60] Such a statutory provision may be exclusive in some states; if so, no indemnification of directors and officers will be permitted outside the statute's provision.[61]

A health care provider also has the power to insure directors against such liability. In fact, any corporation ordinarily has the power to obtain insurance against the liability of a director even beyond the corporation's legal power to indemnify the person.[62]

Antitrust prosecution has been recognized as a very real occupational hazard of corporate directors.[63] The policy underlying both indemnification and insurance provisions has been stated to be "to promote the desirable end that corporate officials will resist what they consider" to be unjustified claims.[64] The larger purpose is to encourage capable individuals "to serve as corporate directors, secure in the knowledge that expenses incurred by them in upholding their honesty and integrity as directors will be borne by the corporation they serve."[65]

Consequently, trustees and directors do not ordinarily face unreasonable risks in executing their functions, but a modest background in antitrust and other legal principles, together with periodic counseling, can reduce their exposure to a minimum.

NOTES

1. Clayton Act § 4, 15 U.S.C. § 15 (1973), permits suits for treble damages by private parties. It also provides for equitable remedies for private plaintiffs. Clayton Act § 16; 15 U.S.C. § 26 (1973);

Allis-Chalmers Mfg. Co. v. White Consol. Indus., 414 F.2d 506 (3d Cir. 1969). The actions also may be cumulative, and the plaintiff in a civil action may enter evidence of any judgment (but not of a consent decree) in a government action as *prima facie* evidence of the violation. Clayton Act § 5(a), 15 U.S.C. § 16(a) (1973).

2. *E.g.*, California Corporations Code § 309(c) (1978), by implication; Model Business Corporation Act § 35, ¶ 2.

3. Hart-Scott-Rodino Antitrust Improvements Act of 1976, Pub. L. 94-435 (1976), provides for these actions by the state as *parens patriae. Cf., State v. Ohio Medical Indemnity, Inc.*, 1976–2 Trade Cases (CCH) ¶ 61,128 (S.D. Ohio 1976); *Nader v. Air Transport Assn of America*, 1977–1 Trade Cases (CCH) ¶ 61,280 (D.C.D.C. 1977) (a consumer has standing to bring an antitrust action where he has suffered a particularized injury). In *Illinois Brick Co. v. Illinois*, 431 U.S. 720, 97 S.Ct. 2061 (1977), in the context of a consumer class action, the Supreme Court held that only a direct purchaser, and not others in the manufacturing or distributing chain, met the Clayton Act § 4 requirement of injury. However, since that decision was announced, there have been continuing Congressional efforts to reverse it legislatively. *See, e.g.*, 898 *Antitrust & Trade Reg. Rep.* (BNA) at A-3 (Jan. 25, 1979). In any event, that decision under the federal statute should not affect the ability of consumers to bring state antitrust claims. *See, e.g., In re Sugar Antitrust Litigation*, 893 *Antitrust & Trade Reg. Rep.* (BNA) at D-4 (Dec. 14, 1978) (claims stated under California's Cartwright Act).

4. *See,* Clayton Act § 8, 15 U.S.C. § 19 (1973). Section 8 is discussed in Wilson, "Unlocking Interlocks," in 45 *Antitrust L. J.* 317 (1976). *See also Boddicker v. Arizona State Dental Assn* , 549 F.2d 626 (9th Cir. 1977) (unnecessary requirements for membership in economically desirable association alleged). Under that definition, the word "commerce" covers trade or commerce among the states, with foreign nations, or between states, territories, or the District of Columbia. In establishing that an interlocking directorate is unlawful, however, it is not necessary to show that the two corporations compete with each other in interstate commerce. *United States v. Sears, Roebuck & Co.*, 111 F. Supp. 614 (S.D.N.Y. 1953).

5. Net worth of the corporation is determined at the end of the fiscal year immediately preceding the election of directors by aggregating capital, surplus, and undivided profits (excluding dividends declared but not paid). Whiting, *Antitrust & the Corporate Executive* (Part I), 47 *Va. L. Rev.* 929, 958 n.114 (1961).

6. Similar fears have been expressed with respect to potential, as well as actual, competition. *See, e.g.*, H.R. 11110, 94th Cong., 1st Sess., Dec. 11, 1975, discussed in Turner, "Interlocks—A Legislative View," 45 *Antitrust L. J.* 331, 332 (1976).

7. *See, e.g.*, Halverson, "Interlocking Directorates—Present Antitrust Enforcement Interest Placed in Proper Analytical Perspective," 21 *Villanova L. Rev.* 393, 394-95, 401-02 (1975-76). Although even indirect interlocks have been argued to be undesirable, the FTC has stated specifically that § 8 of the Clayton Act does not apply to: interlocking directorates between corporate buyers and sellers; competing corporations having directors on the board of a customer or supplier; two competing corporations having a director on the board of a third corporation that is in competition with the two other corporations; interlocks through officers and stockholders as well as other indirect ties; or corporations that are potential competitors. *Report of the Federal Trade Commission on Interlocking Directorates* (1950).

8. Such immunity is far from clear in view of the holding in *Hospital Building Co. v. Trustees of Rex Hosp.*, 425 U.S. 738 (1976).

9. *United States v. Sears, Roebuck & Co.*, 111 F.Supp. 614 (S.D.N.Y. 1953) (such a requirement would ignore the preventive nature of § 8).

10. *Id.*

11. *Id.*

12. *United States v. W. T. Grant Co.*, 345 U.S. 629 (1953).

13. *See United States v. Sears, Roebuck & Co.*, 111 F.Supp. 614 (S.D.N.Y. 1953) (injunction against corporation); Clayton Act § 11, 15 U.S.C. § 21 (1973) which permits the FTC to order a corporation to "rid itself of the directors" who are selected contrary to § 8.

14. *Schectman v. Wolfson*, 244 F.2d 537 (2d Cir. 1957). The availability of such derivative actions is discussed in detail in "Stockholders' Remedies for Corporate Injury Resulting From Antitrust Violations," 59 *Mich. L. Rev.* 904 (1961).

15. *See, e.g., National Supply Co. v. Hillman*, 57 F.Supp. 4 (W.D. Pa. 1944).

16. *E.g., United States v. W.T. Grant Co.*, 112 F.Supp. 336 (S.D.N.Y. 1952), *aff'd*, 345 U.S. 629 (1953) (civil action); *cf., Schechtman v. Wolfson*, 141 F.Supp. 453 (S.D.N.Y. 1956), *aff'd*, 244 F.2d 537 (2d Cir. 1957) (shareholders' derivative suit). The only case under Section 8 to reach the Supreme Court, *United States v. W. T. Grant Co.*, involved the propriety of such a dismissal by the district court over the objection of the government. 345 U.S. 629 (1953). *Dierks Forests, Inc., & Pickering Lumber Corp.*, [1959-1960 FTC Transfer Binder] Antitrust & Trade Reg. Rep. (BNA) ¶ 29,437 (1961); *Booth-Kelly Lumber Co.*, [1959-1960 FTC Transfer Binder] Antitrust & Trade Reg. Rep. (BNA) ¶ 28,388 (1958) (administrative actions).

17. The common law obligations of officers and directors of a corporation to shareholders and to the corporation are set by the law of the state of incorporation. *Childs v. RIC Group, Inc.*, 331 F. Supp. 1078 (D. Ga. 1970), *aff'd mem.*, 447 F.2d 1407 (5th Cir. 1971). *See, e.g.*, California Corporation Code § 309(a) (1978). *See also* New York Business Corporation Law § 717 (1978); Michigan Comp.L.Anno. § 450.1541 (1973); Delaware Code Anno. § 141 (1976); Model Business Corporation Act § 35, discussed in *Corporate Directors Guidebook*, 32 *Bus. L.*, 5, 14-15, 41-47 (1976). Definition of what is in the corporation's "best interest" is complicated by conflicting legal mandates both to contain costs and to be competitive, particularly to the extent the evaluation of the "best interests" is judged in noneconomic terms.

18. *E.g.*, California Corporations Code § 309(b) (1978); Delaware Corporation Code Anno. § 141(e) (1976); Model Business Corporation Act § 43 ¶ 2.02(1)(c).

19. The phrase "corporate interlocks" also arises where the focus is not on competition between one corporation and another, but rather on the dealings between purchaser and supplier corporations that share a common board member. This situation raises issues of self-dealing or of usurpation of corporate opportunity outside the scope of the present inquiry, but are discussed in, *e.g., Shlensky v. South Parkway Bldg. Corp.*, 19 Ill. 2d 268, 166 N.E.2d 793 (1960) (where self-dealing is alleged, the burden is on the challenged directors to show the fairness of the transaction); *Geddes v. Anaconda Copper Mining Co.*, 254 U.S. 590 (1921); *United States v. Delaware, Lackawanna & Western Ry. Co.*, 238 U.S. 516 (1915); Carrington and McElroy, "Doctrine of Corporate Opportunity as Applied to Officers, Directors and Stockholders of Corporations," 14 *Bus. L.* 957 (1959).

20. Stock acquisitions or mergers can, of course, be antitrust violations. This would appear to be an area of particular exposure for trustees and directors who ordinarily make such major decisions. *Allis-Chalmers Mfg. Co. v. White Consol. Indus.*, 414 F.2d 506 (3d Cir. 1969), relying on Clayton Act § 7, 15 U.S.C. § 18 (1973). *See also United States v. Northwest Industries, Inc.*, 1969 Trade Cases (CCH) ¶ 72,853 (N.D.Ill.) (antitrust suit by Justice Department to block a proposed merger).

21. *E.g., Donsco, Inc. v. Casper Corp.*, 587 F.2d 602 (3d Cir. 1978) (a corporate officer is personally liable for authorizing and approving acts of unfair competition as a participant in an unlawful act). Under New York law, illegal acts committed by directors of a corporation may be a breach of fiduciary duty even if they result in a benefit to the corporation. *Miller v. American Tel. & Tel.*, 507 F.2d 759 (3d Cir. 1974).

22. Sherman Act §§ 1, 3, 15 U.S.C. §§ 1, 3 (1973); Clayton Act § 14, 15 U.S.C. § 24 (1973).

23. Clayton Act § 14, 15 U.S.C. § 24 (1973). *See also* 18 U.S.C. § 2 (1973).

24. *Cf., Tillman v. Wheaton-Haven Recreation Ass'n,* 517 F.2d 1141 (a corporate director who actually votes for the commission of a tort is personally liable, even though the wrongful act was performed in the name of the corporation). An antitrust action is one in tort. *Northwestern Oil Co. v. Socony-Vacuum Oil Co.,* 138 F.2d 967 (7th Cir. 1943).

25. At least under Pennsylvania law. *Metzger v. Am. Food Management,* 389 F. Supp. 469 (W.D.Pa. 1975) (securities fraud). *See also, Bellis v. Thal,* 373 F.Supp. 120 (E.D.Pa. 1974), *aff'd mem.,* 510 F.2d 969 (5th Cir. 1975) (where a corporate fiduciary approves, acquiesces in, or conceals a breach of duty by another, both are liable under Pennsylvania law).

26. *See United States v. Morgan,* 118 F.Supp. 621, 694 (S.D.N.Y. 1953) (citing the potential for head-on conflict "between the SEC on one hand and the Antitrust Division of the Department of Justice on the other"). *Cf.* Wild, "Antitrust and the Securities Industry: Lessons from the Shipping Industry," 55 *Cornell L. Rev.* 96 (1969) (such collisions can occur when a regulatory agency permits a merger or uniform rate setting in order to improve service in an industry).

27. *See* discussion of *Hospital Building Co. v. Trustees of Rex Hosp. infra.*

28. 425 U.S. 738 (1976).

29. 370 U.S. 405 (1962).

30. Sherman Act § 1, 15 U.S.C. § 1 (1973). *See also* Clayton Act § 14, 15 U.S.C. § 24 (1973).

31. 370 U.S. at 416.

32. The entire *Wise* opinion consists of a discussion of the reasons—legislative, logical, and policy—for the imposition of such liability.

33. Although this discussion refers throughout to "shareholders," members of a nonprofit or not-for-profit corporation can bring similar suits in the form of derivative actions even where there is no explicit provision for such an action in the statute. *E.g., Valle v. North Jersey Automobile Club,* 125 N.J.Super.Ct. 302, 310 A.2d 518, 521 (1973). *See also* note 49 below.

34. *Thomson v. Mortgage Investment Co.,* 99 Cal. App. 205, 212, 278 P. 468, 471 (1929).

35. Although normally the corporation's right can be enforced only by it or by a shareholder in a derivative action, in the event of corporate insolvency, a trustee in bankruptcy may bring such action. *In re Brunner Air Compressor Corp.,* 287 F. Supp. 256 (N.D.N.Y. 1968).

36. *E.g., Sutter v. Gen. Petroleum Corp.,* 28 Cal. 2d 525, 170 P.2d 898 (1946).

37. The logic of this analysis is discussed in Marsh, *California Corporation Law and Practice* § 14.28. *Cf., Ramsburg v. Am. Inv. Co.,* 231 F.2d 333 (7th Cir. 1956). There is some indication that a derivative action may not be used to right an alleged violation of the antitrust laws. *E.g., Hand v. Kansas City S. Ry. Co.,* 55 F.2d 333 (7th Cir. 1931). In any case, however, the same facts supporting a derivative suit would supply a cause of action under the Clayton Act. *Graham v. Allis-Chalmers Mfg. Co.,* 40 Del.Ch. 335, 182 A.2d 328 (1962), *aff'd,* 41 Del. Ch. 78, 188 A.2d 125 (1963).

38. *See, e.g.,* California Corporations Code § 800 (1978); New York Business Corporations Law § 627 (1978). Federal Rules of Civil Procedure, rule 23.1, 28 U.S.C. (1978), sets similar criteria but does not require the posting of security. The federal rule explicitly provides for derivative actions to be brought by members of nonprofit corporations, as does the New York statute. *See also* Model Business Corporation Act § 49 (1976), and note 44 below.

39. *E.g.,* California Corporations Code § 800(d) (1978), which provides that the security required will not exceed an aggregate of $50,000 for all defendants.

40. *Landy v. F.D.I.C.,* 486 F.2d 139 (3d Cir. 1973), *cert. denied,* 416 U.S. 960 (1974) (generally, responsibility for determining whether a corporation should seek to vindicate an alleged cause of action for damages through court action is a matter of internal management for the board of direc-

tors). *See also, Swanson v. Traer,* 249 F.2d 854 (7th Cir. 1957); *Findley v. Garrett,* 109 Cal. App. 2d 166, 240 P. 2d 421 (1952). *Contra, Groel v. United Electric Co.,* 70 N.J. Eq. 616, 61 A. 1061 (N.J.Ch. 1905).

41. *Loeb v. Berman,* 217 Cal. 716, 20 P. 2d 685 (1933). The same rationale may account in part for the rule that a derivative action may not be dismissed or settled without the approval of the court.

42. *Loeb v. Berman,* 217 Cal. 716, 20 P. 2d 685 (1933).

43. California Corporations Code § 317 (1978).

44. *E.g., Wickersham v. Crittenden,* 106 Cal. 329, 39 P. 603 (1865).

45. *Jacuzzi v. Jacuzzi Bros., Inc.,* 243 Cal. App.2d 1, 36, 52 Cal. Rptr. 147, 171 (1966); *Otis & Co. v. Pennsylvania Ry. Co.,* 57 F. Supp. 680 (E.D. Pa. 1944).

46. *See Garner v. Wolfinbarger,* 430 F. 2d 1093 (5th Cir. 1970); ABA Code of Professional Responsibility DR 5-105 (1977).

47. *See, e.g.,* "Panel Discussion: Interlocking Directorates," 45 *Antitrust L. J.* 352, 353 (1976).

48. *See,* Halverson, "Should Interlocking Director Relationships Be Subject to Regulation and, If So, What Kind?" 45 *Antitrust L. J.* 341, 348–51 (1976).

49. That concern has been expressed particularly by the SEC in its many statements on the responsibilities of corporate directors. *See, e.g.* Proposed Rules Resulting from Corporate Governance Hearings, Secs. Exch. Act Rel. No. 34-14970 (July 18, 1978). Such increased concern with internal oversight and corporate accountability call into question judicial statements such as the one in *Graham v. Allis-Chalmers,* 41 Del.Ch. 78, 118 A.2d 125 (S.Ct. 1963), absolving directors of derivative liability for antitrust violations in the absence of any actual knowledge of those violations, and rejecting plaintiffs' contention that "they should have put into effect a system of watchfulness which would have brought said misconduct to their attention. . . ." 188 A.2d at 130. Today, a court might well require instituting such a "system of watchfulness."

50. 281 F. Supp. 837 (S.D.N.Y. 1968), *rev'd on other grounds,* 426 F. 2d 32 (2d Cir. 1970), *aff'd mem.,* 404 U.S. 548 (1972).

51. Such an orientation is recommended by the *Corporate Directors Guidebook,* prepared by the Subcommittee on Functions and Responsibilities of Corporate Directors of the Committee on Corporate Laws, Section of Corporation, Banking and Business Law of the American Bar Association, and published in 32 *Bus. L.* 5, 18 (1976).

52. *See Cott Beverage Corp. v. Canada Dry Ginger Ale,* 146 F. Supp. 300 (S.D.N.Y. 1956), *appeal dismissed,* 245 F.2d 795 (2d Cir. 1957) (outside directors can be proper parties defendant to a corporate treble damage suit).

53. *Beard v. Aschenbach Mem. Hosp. Assn.,* 170 F. 2d 859, 862 (10th Cir. 1948) (Under Kansas law, bad judgment not amounting to bad faith or gross negligence does not warrant the renditions of a personal judgment against directors). *Cf., Abbey v. Control Data Corp.,* 460 F. Supp. 1242 (D.C. Minn. 1978) (the fact that a suit involves questions arising under the federal securities law does not make application of the business judgment rule inappropriate).

54. California Corporations Code § 317(b) (1978). The California statute was modeled on the Delaware one, *see,* Delaware General Corporation Law § 145 (1976). The Delaware statute is analyzed in detail in E. Folk, *The Delaware General Corporation Law* 95-104 (1972). An extensive if somewhat dated discussion of this area is contained in G. Washington and J. Bishop, *Indemnifying the Corporate Executive* (1963). These authors qualify the problem as one of deciding "[w]ho shall bear the risks of litigation . . ." *Id.* at 1. Indemnification is not a one-way proposition, and directors can be required to indemnify the corporation for fines, civil damages, and attorneys' fees for which it becomes liable as a result of directors' illegal acts that constitute antitrust violations. *Cf., Wilshire Oil Co. v. Riffe,* 409 F.2d 1277 (10th Cir. 1969) (acts of employees). *See also* Anno., *Right of*

Corporation to Indemnity for Civil or Criminal Liability Incurred by Employee's Violation of Antitrust Laws, 37 A.L.R. 3d 1355.

55. California Corporations Code § 317(c) (1978); Delaware Corporations Code Anno. § 145(c) (1976). The fact that a director acted in good faith or with good intentions is not a defense to an antitrust action, *American-Amusement Co. v. Ludwig*, 82 F. Supp. 265 (D. Minn. 1949), so such indemnification provides important protection for the well-intentioned director.

56. California Corporations Code § 317(c)(1) (1978).

57. California Corporations Code § 317(c)(1) (1978).

58. California Corporations Code § 317(c)(2) (1978).

59. California Corporations Code § 317(e),(h) (1978).

60. California Corporations Code § 317(f) (1978).

61. *But see*, Delaware General Corporation Law § 145(f) (1976), which states explicitly that its provisions are not exclusive of other rights under any "bylaw, agreement, vote of shareholders or disinterested directors or otherwise."

62. *E.g.*, California Corporations Code § 317(i) (1978).

63. *See* the famous dissent of Judge Van Voorhis in *Schwartz v. Gen. Aniline & Film Corp.*, 279 App.Div. 996, 998, 112 N.Y.S. 146, 150 (1952), *aff'd*, 305 N.Y. 395, 113 N.E.2d 533 (1953) (antitrust prosecution is "an occupational hazard to the officers and directors of large corporations as truly as falling from a ladder is an occupational hazard to a painter or carpenter").

64. *Essential Enterprises Corp. v. Automatic Steel Products, Inc.*, 39 Del. Ch. 371, 379, 164 A. 2d 437, 441–42 (Ch. 1960).

65. *Mooney v. Willys-Overland Motors, Inc.*, 204 F.2d 888, 898 (3d Cir. 1953).

Case Index

B

Ballard v. Blue Shield of Southern West Virginia, Inc., 117, 141, 185

Bartholomew v. Virginia Chiropractors Association, Inc., 132, 144, 185

Bates v. State Bar of Arizona, 59, 69, 131

Baum v. Investors Diversified Serv., Inc., 202, 210

Beard v. Aschenbach Memorial Hospital Association, 220, 225

Bell v. Georgia Dental Association, 112, 140

Bellis v. Thal, 216, 224

Belliston v. Texaco, Inc., 135, 136, 146

Benell v. City of Virginia, 155

Berkey Photo, Inc. v. Eastman Kodak Co., 11, 22

Biddle Purchasing Co. v. Federal Trade Commission, 205, 211

Blalock v. Ladies Professional Golf Association, 119, 141

Blank v. Palo Alto-Stanford Hospital Center, 150-152, 153, 154, 155, 166

Blue Cross of Virginia v. Commonwealth of Virginia, 132, 144

Board of Trade of City of Chicago v. United States, 4-5, 21, 159

Boddicker v. Arizona State Dental Association, 110, 140, 213-214, 222

Bogus v. American Speech and Hearing Association, 112-113

Borden Co. v. Federal Trade Commission, 201, 210

Brown Shoe Co. v. United States, 101, 105

Burch v. Goodyear Tire and Rubber Co., 15, 22

C

California Motor Transport Co. v. Trucking, Unlimited, 45, 46, 48, 68, 139

Cantor v. Detroit Edison Company, 59-60, 65, 111, 182

Cement Manufacturers Protective Association v. United States, 136, 146

Central Bank of Clayton v. Clayton Bank, 49, 68

Central Ice Cream Co. v. Golden Rod Ice Cream Co., 194, 208

Charlotte Telecasters, Inc. v. Jefferson-Pilot Corp., 43, 67

Chessick Clinic, P.A. v. Jones, 159, 170

Childs v. RIC Group, Inc., 215, 223

Citizen Publishing Co. v. United States, 97, 105

City of Fairfax v. Fairfax Hospital Association, 61-63, 79

City of Lafayette, Louisiana v. Louisiana Power and Light Co., 60-61, 65, 69, 199, 209

Clausen & Sons, Inc. v. Theo. Hamm Brewing Co., 202, 210

Community Blood Bank of Kansas City Area v. Federal Trade Commission, 15, 22

Corleto v. Shore Memorial Hospital, 163, 170

Cott Beverage Corporation v. Canada Dry Ginger Ale, 220, 225

Council for Employment and Economic Energy Use v. WHDH Corp., 126, 142

Cowan v. Gibson, 167-168

Cowen v. New York Stock Exchange, 119, 141

Crawford v. American Title Insurance Company, 181

Crown Zellerbach Corp. v. Federal Trade Commission, 100, 105

Index

A

About the Author

Martin J. Thompson is a partner in the Los Angeles based law firm of Memel, Jacobs, Pierno & Gersh, where he specializes in antitrust and health care counseling and litigation. Mr. Thompson received his Juris Doctorate degree from the University of California at Berkeley where he was an Associate Editor of the California Law Review. He received an A.B. in Economics from the University of California at Davis. He has previously lectured to various professional groups on the subject of antitrust in the health care industry and has provided articles on the subject to other academic and professional organizations.

Date Due